SCOLIOSIS
HOPE

HOW NEW APPROACHES
TO TREATMENT ARE
TRANSFORMING LIVES

DR. TONY NALDA

Scoliosis Hope
How New Approaches to Treatment Are Transforming Lives

Copyright © 2019 by Dr. Tony Nalda

ISBN 978-0-578-49836-2

CONTENTS

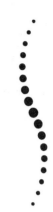

INTRODUCTION

My Scoliosis Story

SINCE I WAS VERY young, I felt drawn to a career in medicine because of my belief in helping others. But I didn't always want to be a chiropractor. In fact, my dream was to become an MD. My course was altered in my teenage years when my life was affected significantly by debilitating migraines.

I was an athletic kid who loved participating in sports, but I had to miss huge portions of my sophomore and junior years of high school, which prevented me from participating in the activities I loved. Back then, there was no such thing as a good day for me. I never knew how my head would feel, and the best I could hope for was a bad day instead of a *really* bad day. My migraines also prevented me from studying and performing up to my potential in my classes. It was awful.

Fortunately, I was able to receive treatment from a chiropractor. I wasn't sure what to expect at first, but by the time I had received a handful of treatments, I knew it was helping me considerably. Even my very first treatment, which wasn't pleasant, provided notable relief. Chiropractic reduced the pain associated with my migraines and virtually eliminated them from my life.

Thanks to this experience and the profound effect it had on my ability to enjoy life, I knew that I wanted to become a chiropractor.

Chiropractic and Scoliosis—A New Way to Treat the Condition

Fast forward to several years later—I found myself operating a highly successful chiropractic practice, treating fifteen hundred patients every week. I was helping lots of people and had established myself as an authority in my field. And yet I had been unable to provide the relief I knew was possible for my scoliosis patients.

In my training, I was taught that there's very little that can be done as a chiropractor to treat scoliosis. The conventional wisdom I received told me that all I could do was manage it and keep it from progressing. One of my young scoliosis patients was not responding favorably to the treatment, and it saddened me to know that the techniques I had learned were not helping her. I wasn't willing to accept this, so I started researching alternative forms of treatment.

I learned that there was, in fact, a chiropractic approach to treating scoliosis that involved more than just adjusting. I traveled with my patient and watched her receive alternative chiropractic treatments for two weeks. This incredibly detailed level of care improved her life and fostered improvements in her condition. Her life was changed—and so was mine.

I realized that I needed to learn new approaches in order to provide relief and improvement to my scoliosis patients. I saw the results firsthand, and I knew I could provide similar relief—not only to my scoliosis patients, but also to *all* of my chiropractic patients—by educating myself on alternative treatments.

Throughout this book, you may notice that I occasionally refer to myself as a *scoliosis chiropractor*. What do I mean by that? Beyond my college degree, I've completed rigorous additional trainings and received certifications outside those typically achieved by chiropractors.

These days, the chiropractic care I provide to scoliosis patients doesn't just address the symptoms; it addresses the issue at the root, just like my migraines were finally relieved by treating my spinal misalignment. No longer do I simply manage my patients' scoliosis. I help them improve their condition, making it possible for them to develop greater strength and functionality.

My goal with this book is to open up a world of possibilities for scoliosis patients and their families. Through my experiences treating patients and watching them improve, I've learned a lot about the condition. I understand what it means to live with scoliosis, and I also know what it's like to overcome the effects of the condition through treatments that aren't as well-known as they should be.

I've also learned quite a bit about the misinformation and misconceptions that people affected by scoliosis must wade through. It's a confusing, intimidating landscape for patients and their family members. I want to end the confusion, demystify the condition, and provide hope.

Throughout this book, I will share stories, insights, and facts that will help you understand the truth about scoliosis. I will also describe an alternative path for those who may feel stuck on a road that leads to surgery and a life of potential complications. It doesn't have to be this way!

There's hope for those with scoliosis who want to lead healthy, active, and meaningful lives. They don't need to be defined by their condition. In fact, they can thrive, become stronger, and act as beacons for the truth about scoliosis. It's my hope that this book will serve as a catalyst.

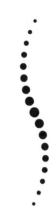

CHAPTER ONE

Defining Scoliosis

What Is Scoliosis? An Introduction to a Confusing Condition

IF YOU ASK THE average person, "What's scoliosis?" they may recall a fuzzy memory of the school nurse visiting their health or gym class. The nurse would ask each student to remove or lift their shirt and bend forward for an examination of the back.

For most people, this scoliosis screening—known as the Adams forward bend test—represents the entirety of their familiarity with the condition. Perhaps they understand, on a basic level, that scoliosis has something to do with the curvature of the spine. But it remains largely mysterious and misunderstood, even among those with friends or family members who must cope with the condition.

Have you been diagnosed with scoliosis recently? Or has someone close to you received a scoliosis diagnosis? If so, you're probably wading through quite a bit of information and advice, unsure of what it all means.

What are the next steps?

What are the most effective treatment options?

Can a person live a normal, active life with scoliosis?

Scoliosis Demystified

One of my goals as a leading expert on scoliosis is to demystify the condition so people with the condition and their loved ones can move forward confidently. The truth is that a scoliosis diagnosis doesn't have to relegate anyone to a life of limitations. People are living rich, full lives with scoliosis, and a number of innovative, noninvasive treatment options have revolutionized the way health-care professionals help their scoliosis patients.

I think it's important to understand the possibilities for positive, transformational outcomes after a scoliosis diagnosis. But first, I want to focus on the big, important question at hand:

What Is Scoliosis?

The Facts about Scoliosis

Essentially, scoliosis is defined as a sideways curvature of the spine, coinciding with spinal rotation. I like to describe it as a 3-D condition, which means that it must be considered in a manner that goes beyond the story that a traditional, two-dimensional X-ray would tell. This is critically important because when the condition is treated in a strictly 2-D manner, it can actually lead to setbacks and further complications. The spine does not simply bend forward or backward, left or right; it bends and curves and rotates in multiple directions.

Cases range from mild (up to a twenty-five-degree curve) to severe (a curve of forty degrees or more), and are progressive, which means that if scoliosis is left untreated, the degree of severity worsens over time.

The causes of scoliosis are, unfortunately, not very well understood. Experts have identified some causes, such as the following:

- cerebral palsy and muscular dystrophy (neuromuscular scoliosis)
- accidents (traumatic scoliosis)
- a defect in the spine such as hemivertebra (congenital scoliosis)
- a result of spinal degeneration (degenerative scoliosis)

However, the majority of scoliosis cases are *idiopathic*—basically, there's no single, known cause. Rather, scoliosis is caused by a host of factors that contribute to its development and progression.

Scoliosis is also probably more common than you think, as well. Consider these facts:

- Estimates indicate that there are more than four million scoliosis cases in the United States alone (National Scoliosis Foundation, 2018).
- Among school-age children, scoliosis is the most common spinal deformity (Chiro & Osteo, 2005).
- Children with scoliosis make more than 440,000 doctor office visits, 133,300 hospital visits and over 17,000 emergency room visits each year (HCUP-AHRQ, 2011).
- Nearly 230,000 adults were hospitalized with scoliosis in 2011 alone. The cost for these hospitalizations was approximately $15.44 million. (BAJB, 2011).
- Scoliosis accounts for 20 percent of all cases of spinal deformity in the United States (BAJB, 2011).

These numbers are even more surprising when you consider that they only describe the number of *diagnosed* scoliosis cases. If you account for those who have scoliosis but have not been diagnosed, the rates are much higher.

Scoliosis affects people from all sectors of the socioeconomic spectrum, and it may be diagnosed at any age. That being said, the most common age of diagnosis is between ten and eighteen, which happens to be the most crucial time for treatment. That's because it's also the age when progression of the condition tends to happen, due to the fact that adolescent bodies grow rapidly in this transitional period.

Typical Treatments for Scoliosis

The traditional approach to scoliosis treatment has been well established. Typically, patients receive a diagnosis, followed by observation and a fitting for a prefabricated brace, with the Boston Brace being the most common. Bracing is done to hold the spine in a straighter alignment, with the goal of preventing the curve from worsening. Sometimes a physical therapy regimen is also prescribed to address pain or imbalances, but this is extremely rare under the traditional treatment model. Additionally, patients often seek chiropractic care on their own (they're seldom referred to chiropractors by traditional scoliosis treatment experts). This may or may not provide relief, depending upon the chiropractor's approach. Ultimately, the traditional approach to scoliosis treatment leads patients down the path to surgery if the curvature continues to progress.

Surgery for scoliosis is performed to stop the progression of the condition through spinal fusion. Outcomes are considered successful when the progression of the condition has ceased. Unfortunately, surgical success doesn't always lead to a healthy body.

Traditional treatments for scoliosis are, in fact, limited in many ways. These methods can be effective, but they tend to focus more on treating a condition than helping a person become more active and functional. What's more, surgery can be prohibitively expensive, and once it has been performed, can leave patients with far fewer options than before.

The Functional Approach to Scoliosis Treatment

When I meet patients, I often see confusion and frustration on their faces before they even utter a single word. They come to me because they've tried the traditional approaches to treating scoliosis, or they're determined to avoid expensive, risky surgeries. People come to me afraid that they will have to make major changes to their lifestyles. They're so caught up in the language of limitation that they fail to see what's possible.

When I was a teenager, my lifestyle was severely limited by excruciating migraines. I was unable to participate in the sports and activities I loved, and I felt resigned to a life of managing and coping instead of achieving my goals. Thankfully, I was able to receive the type of treatment that allowed me to function and live my life to its fullest potential.

My point is that I've been in the same boat so many of my current patients find themselves in, and I understand the frustration and confusion. I challenged the notion that care and treatment should be limiting and focused on simply managing a condition. I knew that it must be possible to treat scoliosis with an approach designed to make life richer and more fulfilling.

My approach to scoliosis treatment focuses on function and the idea that the condition shouldn't stand in the way of one's ambitions and goals. I believe treatment should be patient-centered, which means that people come first. Always. My approach aims to increase mobility and balance, and it engages patients in a way that gets them excited about participating in the process of improving. Most importantly, the functional approach I believe in works—98 percent of my patients experience noticeable relief or improvement after just two weeks!

Scoliosis Progression Demystified

"Will my scoliosis progress?" This is probably the most common question I get asked, and this question requires the most clarifying. When I see patients, all I hear from them is confusion regarding their scoliosis. This happens especially after their curve has progressed. The story I hear all the time from parents is that it seemed to happen overnight, or they didn't know it could get this bad when they were told to watch and wait.

When I see adults who are now suffering with scoliosis, they're normally shocked at how their curve has progressed and confused about why they were told not to worry about it. As a parent of a child with scoliosis or a person with scoliosis, you deserve the facts regarding this process. Understanding the risk factors associated with scoliosis progression can help you make the right decisions.

In fact, this question is really two questions, "Will my curve get worse?" which is normally immediately followed by, "How much worse?" The risk of progression and degree of curve is what influences most of the decision making when treating a patient with scoliosis.

With the traditional approach, the only real treatment that attempts curve reduction is an invasive surgery. This is why most patients are left in the dark regarding the natural progression of scoliosis. However, if I were to answer this without an explanation, then my answer would be, yes, at some point your scoliosis is more than likely going to progress—but no one can tell you exactly how much.

I know this may be vague, but let me further explain by giving you the facts. First fact: the number one risk factor for rapid progression in scoliosis is growth. The faster the growth, the greater the risk of progression. This explains why I hear from parents that it seemed to happen overnight. If parents were just informed that, during puberty, when their child goes through rapid growth, this is the time that progression can occur and they should monitor their child more closely.

This accelerated growth spurt, unfortunately, can be very fast. This spurt normally starts for girls, around eleven years of age and for boys around thirteen years of age. This is normally the pinnacle of risk for rapid progression of scoliosis, but it's impossible to predict exactly when that will happen for each person. Progression due to growth is possible until a child reaches skeletal maturity.

Second fact: puberty isn't a point in time, but a phase of around two years. The curve is at risk for progression until the entire growth phase has been completed. Many doctors will tell girls that once they got their cycle they need not worry anymore, which is totally false.

Third fact: young to middle-aged adult curves do progress, but normally much slower than growing kids. When I was in chiropractic college, I was taught that adult curves don't progress. In fact, I know this is still taught today *and* is false. The progression that happens for a young adult is normally slow. This is due to gravity, which is more likely to lead to compression and pain. Since this progression is slower, the progression can be unnoticeable. Let's say it's only one degree a year. One degree a year isn't a lot, but over ten, twenty, thirty years, it can really add up.

Fourth fact: the bigger the curve, the greater risk of progression. This is true for kids and adults. So, for kids, the younger the child and the bigger the curve, the greater risk for a rapid-phase progression. For adults, as curves get bigger, it's more likely they can continue to get bigger.

Fifth fact: adults in later stages of life can experience faster progression. This can be a frightening fact, but as people age with scoliosis, the curved spine can lead to asymmetrical degenerative changes within the spine itself. This leads to increased rate of progression post forty to fifty years of age, and it can really start to pick up past sixty years of age.

Sixth fact: for women, menopause can lead to an increased rate of scoliosis progression. It has been noticed that there's an increased rate of progression during and after menopause. This is thought to be because of bone mineral loss that can occur during menopause.

Seventh fact: no one can tell how many degrees a curve will progress. This is the really frustrating part with scoliosis, that the degree of progression can be so varied from one person to the next. Two children of the same age, with ten-degree curves—even though they looked the same at ten degrees, one can progress to sixty degrees, while the other will only progress to twenty-five degrees. The same thing is true for adult cases. Some progress faster. Some progress slower.

Let's look at what can happen and why I say watching and waiting can be one of the worst recommendations ever given.

First, for an adolescent. An eleven-year-old girl is diagnosed with a twenty-degree curve. Her doctor says, "Don't worry about it. It's a mild scoliosis." The doctor prescribes watch-and-wait and tells her to return in six months. The very next day, she initiates her pubertal growth spurt. At this time, curves can progress fast. She returns six months later and now has a forty-degree curve. The doctor now recommends surgery, and the parents are shocked.

The traditional treatment doctor will say, "We didn't know it would progress, so why do anything?"

I say, "Sure, that may be true. But reducing a twenty-degree curve to ten degrees isn't harmful. Risking a curve progressing to forty degrees is."

Now, for adults. A twenty-one-year-old woman has a twenty-degree curve with mild lower back pain. She's given pain pills, told not to worry because it's a mild scoliosis. Let's say she's only progressing half a degree a year. At sixty, she now has a surgical-level curve and wonders why she wasn't told when she was twenty-one to do something. If she's progressing one degree a year, now it's a sixty-degree curve. If she's progressing two degrees a year, it's a hundred-degree curve!

Lastly, let's look at a juvenile, a six-year-old boy with a fifteen-degree curve. Again, the doctor says *mild scoliosis, watch and wait*, and the patient is told to return in a year. He is growing slowly at this time, so it may only progress five degrees over this entire year. Now, being seven years old, they repeat his initial recommendation—watch and wait and return next year.

The patient returns at eight years of age, and now it's twenty-five degrees. Again, very little progression, and he's told to return next year. At nine, now the curve is thirty degrees. The patient is told to wear a Boston Brace for twenty-three hours a day—and all it can do is keep the curve from getting worse. If it continues to get worse, the patient will need surgery.

Remember, this child's pubertal growth spurt is still to come. Therefore, I say that, with juvenile scoliosis, we must reduce the curve before this growth spurt to reduce that risk.

So, progression of scoliosis has periods of rapid progression and periods of slower progression, but more and more data is leading us to understand that, more than likely, scoliosis progression at some level is expected. How much is different for everyone.

Twelve Scoliosis Myths, Busted!

To gain an understanding of what scoliosis *is*, I think it's important to not only define and describe it, but also to also explain what it *is not*.

As a leader on scoliosis and scoliosis treatment, I encounter a number of myths and misconceptions on an almost daily basis. People often come to me confused and scared about the condition, and the research they've done typically contains just as much falsehood as it does truth.

My hope is that people can gain a better, more realistic understanding of scoliosis. I want them to honestly understand what the condition means for both young people and adults. I see far too many people taking the watch-and-wait approach without ever questioning the conventional wisdom they're given. They don't know that effective alternative treatments are available. And they see no reason *not* to believe the myths and misconceptions that surround scoliosis.

Of course, it's impossible, given the sheer number of misconceptions that exist, to bust all of them. But the following scoliosis myths are the ones I discuss with patients most frequently.

Myth #1—"Scoliosis Is Caused by..."

There are a lot of ideas out there regarding the causes of scoliosis—and most of them are wrong!

Carrying a heavy backpack does not cause scoliosis. Nor does participating in certain physical activities. The list goes on and on.

Whenever you hear or read information that purports to know the cause of scoliosis, you should be skeptical. The fact is that the vast majority of scoliosis cases are idiopathic, which means there's no known cause. A multitude of factors contribute to the development of the condition. It's not unlike having a fever, if you think about it. A fever, like scoliosis, is really just a symptom; it's the result of a host of other factors. Even though it's a manifestation of an illness, it's not the illness.

Myth #2—Scoliosis Is Preventable

Again, because we don't know exactly what causes most cases of scoliosis, we can't engage in methods to prevent it from occurring. There's no diet, type of exercise, or lifestyle practice that will stave off the condition. The best we can do is take a proactive approach to treatment once the condition has been diagnosed. Thankfully, treatments like those we provide here at the Scoliosis Reduction Center are highly effective and can often reduce curvatures.

Myth #3—Scoliosis Makes the Body Weak and Frail

An abnormal curvature of the spine does not equate to a decrease in strength or bone density. In fact, people with scoliosis can be just as capable, strong, and fit as anyone else.

Myth #4—Scoliosis Can Cause Organ Failure

One of the more popular scoliosis misconceptions is that the curvature of the spine can press into organs, causing them to fail. This just isn't true. As the spine curves and twists, so does everything else in the body. In most cases, the spine actually curves *away* from the heart and other vital organs.

This being said, scoliosis *can* cause some lung deficiencies, but only when the curve is extremely severe (around eighty degrees, for example), and not because of the spine pushing on the lungs. When taking the watch and wait approach, the spine can tend to become more rigid, which can also lead to lung deficiencies.

Myth #5—Women with Scoliosis Can't Have Children

I've addressed this issue time and time again, but it bears repeating since it's such a commonly accepted piece of misinformation: scoliosis does not prevent conception or a healthy birth. It does not diminish fertility in any way, nor does it increase the possibility of miscarriage. There's no difference between women with scoliosis and women without scoliosis when it comes to the ability to conceive and bear healthy children.

Myth #6—Young People with Scoliosis Can't Participate in Sports

I actually *prefer* it when young people with scoliosis participate in sports and other physical activities. We want them to be active! The stronger, more balanced, and more coordinated they are, the better the results we can get from treatment. However, there are some activities like dance and gymnastics that we would recommend limiting for scoliosis patients. But if a patient is complying with treatment, no limitations are typically placed on them.

Myth #7—Scoliosis Is Always Painful

Yes, scoliosis can cause pain in adult patients, but for young people, pain is usually not a factor. This is because the upward motion of the spine's growth in adolescence actually relieves the pressure that might otherwise cause pain.

The opposite myth—that scoliosis *never* causes pain—is also fairly persistent and equally untrue.

Myth #8—Traditional Bracing Apparatus Can Correct Scoliosis

Traditional bracing apparatus such as the Boston Brace, Milwaukee Brace, or Providence Brace (also known as a nighttime brace) aren't meant to correct abnormal spinal curvatures. They're used to prevent the worsening of the curvature. Ultimately, those who are prescribed traditional scoliosis braces and participate in traditional treatments may continue down a path that leads to surgery.

Myth #9—Children Can Grow Out of Their Curves

This misconception is a symptom of the watch-and-wait approach that's become the standard of treatment. Certainly, there are some curves that will not progress past adolescence, but no one grows out of an abnormal curvature. When you work to reduce the curve, there's no harm done if it ends up not progressing. But when you fail to engage in treatment, you can actually cause tremendous harm.

Truly, the only chance of a curve being grown out of is in the infantile phase. For adolescents or older patients, it's just not possible that the curve will grow straighter.

Myth #10—Scoliosis Curves Remain Static in Adulthood

Doctors and orthopedic specialists will often tell patients that once they're adults, they don't need to worry about the progression of their curvatures. The fact is that curves can continue to progress, even in adulthood, once the body has stopped growing.

Myth #11—Surgery Can Cure Scoliosis

A true scoliosis cure would return the spine's curvature to normal without imposing any other limitations to spinal function, but that's not at all what surgery does. It can relieve pain, stabilize the spine, and restore some function, but it's not a cure, and there's no guarantee that it will create any improvements. Surgery can make the spine straighter, but at the great expense of the consequences of surgical fusion, which always reduces function. It does not address the underlying causes of the condition; in fact, it can cause new problems for the spine.

Myth #12—Chiropractic-Centered Treatment Doesn't Work

This myth is especially popular among scoliosis surgeons, and I understand why they take this position. Providing surgery for scoliosis is their profession and source of income. It's also the treatment approach they truly believe in, even though chiropractic-centered scoliosis treatment has shown itself to be incredibly effective. Therefore, they continue to put patients on the path to surgery, citing the watch-and-wait approach as the only sensible form of treatment.

Truthfully, most surgeons have zero training in the types of conservative treatments that could reduce the impact of scoliosis; they have no idea how to help those who come to them seeking a way to avoid surgery. It's just like how I have no way to help those who come to me seeking surgery—it's just not what I do.

I know better. That's why we see patients from all around the world here at the Scoliosis Reduction Center. Our treatment method is dynamic, comprehensive, proactive—and effective. It actually works to reduce curvatures, restore function, and help people live their best lives.

Nine Surprising Scoliosis Statistics

I believe the best way to understand scoliosis is on a patient-by-patient basis. Each individual is unique, and there are no two scoliosis cases that are exactly alike. Every spine tells its own story, and every patient has their own distinct relationship with the condition. Nevertheless, I think it can be useful to take a broader view of scoliosis from time to time in order to understand the big picture.

In reality, scoliosis affects more than just each individual patient. It affects parents, family members, friends, teachers, coaches, and our entire society.

To help you understand the impact that scoliosis has in our world, here are some surprising statistics from CLEAR Scoliosis Institute that will help you put the condition into perspective.

#1—29,000 Adolescent Surgeries Each Year

Every year in the United States alone, approximately 29,000 scoliosis surgeries are performed on adolescent patients.

Think about that for a moment: 29,000 annual surgeries every year breaks down to an average of nearly eighty surgeries per day—and three every hour! When you consider the cost of surgery and the impact it can have on an adolescent's life, this number is staggering. That's a lot of money and a lot of big changes in the lives of young people and their families.

#2—$92,000 for a Child's Hospital Stay

On average, it costs $92,000 for a child with scoliosis to stay in the hospital.

This number is just the *average* amount for a child's hospital stay when they have scoliosis. In many cases, that figure can rise well above $100,000. This amount is even more surprising when you consider that the national average cost for a child's hospital stay (for all conditions) is $17,500.

#3—Twice the Average Hospital Charge
For adults with scoliosis, the average hospital charge is approximately double the national average.

The average three-day hospital stay for an adult in the United States costs $30,000, according to healthcare.gov. A scoliosis patient can expect to pay $60,000. That's hugely significant. In fact, scoliosis alone accounts for 1.2 percent of all hospital charges each year.

Also, consider the fact that adults with scoliosis are more likely to need long-term medical care than those without the condition. If hospital stays are involved, the costs associated with scoliosis in adults can rise dramatically.

#4—Emergency Room Scoliosis Treatment Is More Common Than You Might Think
Every year in the United States, children with scoliosis make 17,500 emergency room visits, and adults with scoliosis make 74,000 visits.

That's more than 90,000 emergency room visits each year from scoliosis patients alone. Break it down by week, and the number is over 1,750. By day, it's more than 250. Wow. And as you know, costs associated with emergency room visits can be astronomical.

#5—Annual Nonsurgical Costs Up to $14,000
According to estimates, direct costs of nonsurgical care for adults with scoliosis can be as high as $14,000. This number does not include the loss of wages or time from work.

When considering the costs associated with scoliosis treatment, it's natural to single out surgical expenses. But other costs add up in a big way, too.

#6—A Communication Breakdown

Ninety percent of scoliosis patients would like more opportunities to discuss their feelings with health-care professionals.

Scoliosis is more than just a mechanical issue of the spine. It affects patients emotionally, as well, but only 5 percent of people with scoliosis say they have had the opportunity to discuss their feelings with doctors or other health-care providers. The vast majority of patients don't feel like they have adequate communication opportunities with the people they're counting on to help them heal.

#7—Severe Emotional Effects

Scoliosis patients are 40 percent more likely to have experienced suicidal thoughts.

Speaking of emotional effects of scoliosis, they can be quite serious and potentially severe. Patients with scoliosis are more likely to experience suicidal thoughts, which is very troubling. They're also more likely to be concerned about abnormal body development and the strain their condition may have on relationships with their peers.

#8—Scoliosis and Back Pain

Seventy-three percent of individuals with scoliosis report experiencing back pain in the previous year. Only 28 percent of people without scoliosis report back pain.

Scoliosis does not always lead to back pain, but back pain is much more common in people with the condition than in the general public. When people experience back pain, their lives are impacted negatively in multiple ways: they're unable to experience a normal range motion, they can't participate in numerous activities they enjoy, and they become limited in terms of their ability to maintain rich and fulfilling social lives.

#9—"Horrible" and Continuous Pain

Scoliosis patients are twice as likely to report continuous pain as patients without scoliosis. Additionally, 23 percent of those with scoliosis report pain levels described as "distressing," "excruciating," or "horrible," compared to 1.4 percent of people who don't have scoliosis.

Let this one sink in. Physical pain is one of the most challenging aspects of life, and people with scoliosis experience it more frequently, continuously, and horribly than those without scoliosis. When you consider that more than four million people in the United States alone have scoliosis, there are a lot of people out there who live in pain. The effect all this pain has on society shouldn't be taken lightly.

The surprising statistics I've cited here may be alarming, or they may simply seem like everyday reality if you or a loved one lives with scoliosis. Regardless of how these facts make you feel, it's crucial to know that efforts are being made to improve these statistics and—most importantly—enhance the lives of people with the condition.

Is Scoliosis Hereditary?

When a patient or parent learns of a scoliosis diagnosis, they often turn to the family tree in the search for answers. They want information and an explanation for why the condition has developed. They wonder, *Is scoliosis hereditary?*

I can understand what drives patients and parents to seek answers in their genetics.

I wish I could give patients the certainty they crave as they try to understand their condition, but the fact is that scoliosis develops as a result of multiple possible factors. And there's no known cause of scoliosis in 80 percent of cases.

If you're wondering if scoliosis is hereditary, the simple answer is no. It does play a small role in idiopathic cases and could be a larger factor in neuromuscular or congenital cases. But those represent a very small portion of the total number of scoliosis cases. Furthermore, the cause of scoliosis does not necessarily matter in terms of how the condition should be treated most effectively. Unless it's a true congenital case where there's a misshapen spinal bone that could alter treatment, or if there are tumors present, the most effective treatment approach remains the same.

This is a tricky issue, and I want to make sure patients, parents, and readers of this book understand the truth about scoliosis, its development, and how it's caused.

What Does Hereditary Mean?

First of all, I think it's important to understand what *hereditary* means.

In terms of genetics, when a condition is described as hereditary, it means that it was passed down from a parent to their offspring; essentially, the parent possesses a particular defective gene, and the child inherits it.

However, truly hereditary conditions and diseases are extremely rare. The inheritance of defective genes seldom happens in reality. Yes, many conditions arise from genetic predispositions, but this is different from defective genes being passed down and inherited by children.

In the case of scoliosis, most experts agree that there's probably a genetic predisposition. But that doesn't mean that the condition is hereditary. Some people with a genetic predisposition develop the condition. Others do not. Even identical twins experience differing rates of scoliosis development. If one twin has scoliosis, the other may or may not also have it. Or they may have a completely different curvature or Cobb angle measurement.

If scoliosis were truly hereditary, every twin with scoliosis would share the condition in exactly the same manner with their identical brother or sister. And we know that's not the case!

Consider heart disease. If a person comes from a line of people who have dealt with the condition, then they may be more susceptible to it themselves. But they can ward off heart disease through diet, exercise, and healthy lifestyle choices. There are simply too many factors involved to be able to say that genetics is the sole cause. Nothing is written in stone with heart disease, and the same is true with scoliosis.

Genetic Factors and the Root Causes of Scoliosis

Scoliosis isn't hereditary, and there's no single, known gene responsible for the condition. There's a familial connection, though. A genetic predisposition may or may not exist within a family, but family members share much more than just their genes.

Environmental factors also come into play in terms of the development of scoliosis. Families tend to live in the same geographic areas, so those factors may be playing a larger part than genetics. Family members also tend to share things like diet, lifestyle, and even posture. They experience similar stresses. They participate in similar activities, too. There's a lot more going on than just genetics, which is why it's impossible to determine a single cause.

Because family members share so much in common, it's easy to see why people would assume a genetic link when scoliosis develops. But the fact is that the condition arises through a multitude of factors, making it impossible to pin the cause on any single element of a person's life or branch of their family tree.

Five Facts about Scoliosis Causes

The cause of scoliosis is a topic of great debate. If it's not hereditary, then where does it come from? Do people participate in activities that cause the abnormal spinal curvature? Are environmental factors to blame?

I wish I could tell patients and their families the precise cause of scoliosis, but as you'll see, this is impossible. Here are five facts that illustrate why it's so difficult to tie scoliosis to a specific cause:

#1—Less Than 20 Percent of All Scoliosis Cases Have a Known Cause

This fact can be frustrating to reckon with, but it's the truth. Fewer than one in five scoliosis cases can be traced to a specific cause, which leaves most people with the condition wondering how it developed. So, what are the direct causes that *can* be identified? They include the following:

- **Congenital scoliosis,** which develops due to a failure of the bones to form properly, contributing to the abnormal curvature of the spine
- **Neuromuscular scoliosis,** which occurs when a disease like cerebral palsy or muscular dystrophy affects the spine in a way that leads to abnormal curvature
- **Traumatic scoliosis,** which happens as a result of surgeries, accidents or other body traumas that affect the spine adversely

- **Degenerative scoliosis**, which occurs in older individuals whose spinal discs have degenerated, leading to the abnormal spinal curvature

#2—Most Cases of Scoliosis Are Idiopathic

The vast majority—80 percent—of scoliosis cases are described as idiopathic, which means they have no known cause. Basically, it's impossible to determine a single causative source of the condition in more than four out of five patients.

It should be noted that idiopathic doesn't mean there's an absence of a cause; it means that the cause isn't apparent or easily determined. Idiopathic can also indicate a multifactorial causation.

#3—The "Scoliosis Gene" Theory Is Deeply Flawed

As I explained previously in this chapter, it's easy to understand why a genetic explanation for scoliosis would be so satisfying. It would eliminate the mystery and the guesswork about how the condition arose and relieve patients of any nagging feelings that they did something wrong to develop scoliosis.

The truth is that attributing a genetic basis to scoliosis is futile. While it's possible that there may be a genetic predisposition for scoliosis, there's no way to know if a gene will be expressed in the carrier. In other words, someone could be carrying the "scoliosis gene," but it may never result in an actual case of scoliosis. Moreover, someone who is *not* a carrier of the gene could develop scoliosis through some other combination of causative factors.

#4—Scoliosis Almost Always Develops from a Combination of Causes

Although we can't trace a person's scoliosis back to a single cause in the majority of cases, it's clear that most idiopathic scoliosis arises due to a combination of factors, both genetic and environmental. Scoliosis isn't a simple condition; it's quite complex, and it affects different people in different ways. This is why each individual must be evaluated independently to determine the factors that are likely contributing to the development and progression of the condition.

#5—If a Single Cause Were Found, the Nature of Treatment May Not Change

Scoliosis causes are mostly unidentifiable, but that doesn't mean the condition can't be treated effectively. In fact, the approach we take here at the Scoliosis Reduction Center has helped us transform the lives of our patients by reducing curvatures, adding strength, and improving function.

Typically, by the time a person knows they have scoliosis—regardless of the causes—it has become structural within the spine itself. Therefore, the treatment now needs to address this.

We utilize a combination of treatments, including scoliosis-specific chiropractic care, therapy, exercise, and corrective bracing. The cause, if it can be determined, rarely plays in to how we approach the successful treatment of our patients.

I can understand why people become frustrated by the lack of clarity that's available regarding the possible causes of scoliosis. But that frustration shouldn't prevent patients, parents, and loved ones from seeking relief from the condition. When you look at the facts about scoliosis causes, you can take comfort knowing that most people are in the same boat—there's no known single cause! However, we *do* know what works when it comes to treating scoliosis and preventing further progression.

As I mentioned previously, there are two prevailing schools of thought regarding scoliosis treatment. There's the traditional approach, which involves watching, waiting, and, eventually, surgery. There's also the functional approach, which aims to improve strength and flexibility while reducing curvatures, giving patients a better alternative for managing their scoliosis.

I believe strongly in the functional, chiropractic-based approach to scoliosis treatment. Unfortunately, most people go through their scoliosis journeys unaware that there are alternatives to the traditional path. In most cases, patients are told that surgery is inevitable.

The Truth about Scoliosis Surgery

I see patients all the time who come to me feeling hopeless, frustrated, and even angry. They've been told that their only path forward is through scoliosis surgery, which is expensive, risky, and not guaranteed to give them the relief that they've been seeking. I also talk to a lot of parents who are terrified at the prospect of having their son or daughter endure—and recover from—a major surgery. They've been advised to take a wait-and-see approach as their child progresses through adolescence, only to be informed that there's ultimately no alternative to surgery. They wonder what they've been waiting and watching for, and I truly empathize with them.

I believe in taking a patient-centered approach to scoliosis care. For me, it's not about what makes sense administratively or for my business's bottom line. It's about what makes sense for my patients.

Unfortunately, far too many people who deal with scoliosis find themselves moving through a system that seems to neglect their needs. They're unaware of alternatives to the reactive type of care they have received. And when they learn that a more proactive approach exists, they feel betrayed by the traditional medical approach.

The fact is that scoliosis rarely gets better on its own. The traditional wait-and-see approach that's so popular within the medical establishment isn't intended to create improvements, but to see how bad the condition gets over time. That's why so many people find themselves at a crossroads with scoliosis: either get surgery or face the consequences of a condition that only worsens over time. And when they opt for surgery, no one can promise that it will reduce or eliminate pain. No one can promise that it will provide cosmetic improvements. No one can promise that additional surgeries won't be necessary.

Some Scoliosis Surgery Facts

I understand why scoliosis surgery is recommended so often to patients and parents. An invasive, surgical, reactive approach to health care is the name of the game in our culture here in the United States, so it's no surprise that the common approach to scoliosis is guided by the same rationale. The surgical approach also happens to be quite lucrative and administratively beneficial for doctors and hospitals.

This is, of course, the opposite of the patient-centered approach that I prefer.

If you look at scoliosis surgery from the perspective of what's best for the patient, it doesn't make as much sense.

Consider these facts:

- Recovery from scoliosis surgery can take weeks, months, or even years. This is particularly troubling for adolescents and younger individuals who must miss school, extracurricular activities, and other crucial events.
- Except for extreme cases, a medical indication for AIS spinal-fusion surgery does not actually exist (Weiss, 2013).

- Over time, the rate of complications from spinal-fusion surgery increases (Weiss, 2013).
- Evidence for improvements in quality of life after spinal-fusion surgery does not exist. (Weiss, 2013).
- Spinal-fusion surgery for scoliosis is incredibly expensive—the average cost for patients is $113,000 (Spine, 2010).
- When surgery isn't successful in reducing pain or correcting cosmetic appearance, the only treatment option left for surgeons to recommend is additional surgeries.
- Surgery simply transforms a spinal deformity into a lifelong spinal dysfunction, which can lead to disfigurement, pain, and long-term disability.
- Surgery reduces the spine's range of motion, even in those areas that have not been fused.
- Spinal-fusion surgery can also lead to complications such as rod displacement, pseudoarthrosis, infection, and nerve damage (Medical News Today, 2017).

When patients and parents learn these facts after being presented with surgery as their only option, they're often led here to the Scoliosis Reduction Center because they're desperate for alternatives. It's no wonder that so many of them are frustrated!

The Alternative Approach to Scoliosis Surgery

As curves progress, scoliosis surgery is the most likely outcome of the traditional medical approach. Fortunately, a more natural, functional, and proactive approach is available for those who wish to avoid the expense, complications, recovery time, and limitations of surgery.

I believe in a method that works to strengthen the spine and build its ability to function. When scoliosis is treated in this manner, the spine can begin to support itself, avoid the progression of scoliosis, and avoid scoliosis surgery! When needed, a unique combination of active and passive rehabilitation, exercise therapy, and chiropractic care work together in a fully comprehensive treatment approach. Yes, it requires dedication and hard work from both the patient and their provider, but it produces real, tangible results. In fact, about 98 percent of my patients experience noticeable relief in just two weeks.

When patients and parents hear about the successes that have been achieved through this alternative approach, they often wonder why no one told them that there was another way forward. I see the frustration on their faces and hear it in their voices. That's why it's so important to me and my staff to spread the word about what's possible when treatment is handled in a patient-centered fashion.

Scoliosis surgery does not have to be the only choice for those who simply want relief, increased functionality, and a healthy appearance.

Why the Chiropractic-Centered Approach Works

Chiropractic is a well-established health-care profession with roots stretching back more than a hundred years. Chiropractors treat more than thirty-five million adults and children each year in the United States alone (Gallup-Palmer, 2016). 95 percent of those who have sought chiropractic care for neck and/or back pain say it's effective, and according to a recent survey, chiropractic outperforms all other treatments for back pain, including Pilates, deep-tissue massage, and yoga (Consumer Reports, 2012).

Obviously, people believe in chiropractic care and the benefits it provides, particularly when it comes to treating neck and/or back pain. What's not as well understood is the benefit chiropractic can provide for scoliosis patients.

Can a chiropractor heal scoliosis? If you've been doing your research, you have probably come across some promising information and a number of success stories. But the question of whether a chiropractor can heal scoliosis requires an answer more complex than a simple yes or no.

I believe strongly in the efficacy of chiropractic care for the treatment of scoliosis, but I also understand that there's a lot of mystery surrounding the subject.

The chiropractic-centered approach, at its core, is about improving the patient's function while reducing the risk of a condition's progression. It's not meant to hide symptoms, and it's not about waiting for something to get worse. Our chiropractic approach to scoliosis is guided by the goals of improving function and reducing risk.

I want to help you understand the truth about what's possible. A chiropractor with the proper training and approach can work wonders for scoliosis patients, but it's important to understand that chiropractic isn't a magic pill. Moreover, chiropractic works best for scoliosis when it's used in conjunction with other therapies.

Also, there's a big difference between treating someone with scoliosis versus treating someone's scoliosis. Obviously, any chiropractor can treat someone with scoliosis, meaning they can provide adjustments and general chiropractic care. However, it takes a trained chiropractor to effectively treat someone's scoliosis to achieve a reduction.

The Chiropractic Approach to Scoliosis, Explained

Chiropractors with the proper training can do amazing things for their scoliosis patients, but it's important to understand a few critical points about the approach:

- A chiropractor can't *heal* scoliosis, but they can do much more than simply *manage* it.
- By taking the proper approach, the progressive nature of scoliosis can be halted and even reversed.
- The chiropractic approach that's most effective utilizes adjustments in addition to exercise and corrective bracing, as well as active and passive rehabilitation techniques, all of which are determined by the specific needs of the patient and are prescribed accordingly.
- The most effective approach typically requires patients to participate in an intensive program, meaning that they should receive a significant amount of treatment in a short period of time.
- Results from clinical treatment are sustained and augmented by a home-treatment program, individualized for each specific patient.
- This multidisciplinary approach can be difficult to obtain since it uses so many different types of treatment, which is why the Scoliosis Reduction Center has become so popular—we provide patients with access to every facet of treatment.

The chiropractic approach to treating scoliosis works so well because it goes beyond addressing symptoms. It addresses the function and strength of the spine, giving patients the chance to transcend their condition and participate in life fully. Yes, it's intense and it requires a strong commitment from each patient. But the results speak for themselves!

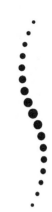

CHAPTER TWO

Life with Scoliosis

A Life of Limitations versus a Life of Possibilities

IN MY OPINION, LIVING with scoliosis shouldn't mean living with excessive boundaries or limitations.

Unfortunately, patients and parents tend to hear scoliosis discussed more often than not in terms of what's *not* possible. They're typically told to be cautious and that surgery—which will alter their bodies and lives in irreversible ways—is the only way to ultimately treat the condition they live with. This creates a scenario in which patients focus so strongly on the promise of future surgery that they forget that they're living life in the here and now.

I believe that scoliosis shouldn't define a person's life. Yes, a person with scoliosis must take their condition under consideration as they make choices in life. But they shouldn't feel as if they're outsiders, or that scoliosis is the characteristic that outshines all others.

In this chapter, I want to continue describing the nature of scoliosis and its effects on people. But I also want to describe the ways in which people can defy the conventional wisdom surrounding the condition.

My goal with this chapter is to truly demystify scoliosis. While there's a lot we don't know about the condition, it's not so mysterious that we can't empathize with those who have it. Scoliosis affects real people—neighbors, friends, family members—and it shouldn't be seen as a rare or exotic condition that can only be corrected through surgical means. Life can be lived in countless healthy and fulfilling ways with scoliosis. And treatment can be just as fulfilling for patients and the people around them who are also affected by scoliosis.

I want to get started with this chapter by describing the three severity levels of scoliosis: mild, moderate, and severe.

Let's get started!

Understanding the Signs of Mild Scoliosis

When it comes to mild scoliosis, the conventional wisdom tells patients and their families to watch and wait. Of course, watching and waiting typically leads to the condition progressing from mild to moderate and, eventually, to severe. I believe that patients have the best chance of treating scoliosis when it's in the earliest, mildest stages. Unfortunately, traditional treatment approaches aren't so proactive. Furthermore, the signs of mild scoliosis can be quite subtle and difficult to discern.

The chiropractic-centered approach to scoliosis treatment can be incredibly effective for mild cases. It can help patients reduce their curvatures and/or halt further progression. Most importantly, it can keep patients off the operating table and away from the surgeon's blade.

The best time to treat scoliosis using the chiropractic-centered approach is when the condition is mild. But before progress can be made, it's important for people to be educated about the signs of mild scoliosis.

Three Severity Levels

Before we begin to talk about the signs of mild scoliosis, I think it's important to understand how doctors describe the different levels of severity.

Experts have come to agreement on the classification of three different severity levels of scoliosis:

- **Mild scoliosis** refers to cases in which the Cobb angle measures at twenty-five degrees or less.
- **Moderate scoliosis** describes cases where the Cobb angle measures between twenty-five and forty degrees.
- **Severe scoliosis** is a term used to describe the condition when Cobb angles measure at forty-plus degrees for adolescents and fifty-plus degrees for adults.

Typically, a Cobb angle needs to measure greater than ten degrees to be diagnosed as scoliosis. When scoliosis is considered mild, the preferred traditional treatment is to watch and wait. But that's actually no treatment at all.

Some doctors will recommend a squeezing type of brace, such as the Boston Brace, once the condition reaches the moderate stage (with a Cobb angle measurement greater than twenty-five degrees, but less than forty). Unfortunately, due to the ineffectiveness of these types of braces, traditional approaches to treatment may not recommend any action until the angle reaches the severe classification. This is very unfortunate! There's a lot that can be done to help patients take control of their condition and avoid the progression of an abnormal spinal curvature.

Initially, mild scoliosis isn't likely to present major obstacles or limitations in terms of its impact on living an active life. But scoliosis isn't a static condition; its nature is to progress and become increasingly severe over time. That is, of course, unless it's treated proactively.

Are you concerned that you or your child may be living with a mild case of scoliosis? Are you unwilling to take the traditional watch-and-wait approach? To help you take the most proactive and helpful approach, here are the signs and factors you should look for.

Clothing Fits Unevenly

It's not uncommon for adolescents to outgrow their clothes quickly. But when the fit of clothing seems uneven or reveals bodily asymmetry, it could be a sign that mild scoliosis is present. Pay attention to the way your child's clothes hang on the body—do sleeves and cuffs appear to be uneven? Do shirt necklines seem to favor one side over the other? An uneven fit isn't proof of scoliosis, but it should cause you to investigate further and determine if other factors are present.

Issues with Balance and Coordination

Yes, teenagers can be awkward, physically. But if an adolescent experiences issues with their balance and/or coordination to a noticeable degree, mild scoliosis may be present. You may also notice problems with proprioception, which is the sense one has of the orientation of the body in its particular environment.

Changes in Gait

The way a person walks can tell you a lot about their physical condition. Often, mild scoliosis reveals itself in the way an adolescent walks. Arms may swing less, and there could be a reduction in the normal counter-rotating motion the body makes in the hips and shoulder. Additionally, asymmetrical motion during the gait could also be a sign of mild scoliosis.

Uneven Posture

Uneven shoulders and hips could be indicators of mild scoliosis. Some other clues may also be present:

- The head isn't centered evenly over the body.
- One arm seems to hang lower than the other.
- Ribs may stick out more on one side than the other.
- While standing, the body appears to tilt to one side.
- One leg appears to be longer than the other.
- One hip appears to sit higher than the other.
- An asymmetrical waist, which is when one side is more curved while the opposite side appears flatter, may become noticeable.
- One shoulder blade protrudes from the body more than the other.
- The space between the arms and torso may appear to be asymmetrical.

Basically, any indication that the body is asymmetrical could be a sign of mild scoliosis.

Pain Is Present

Adolescent scoliosis patients don't experience pain to the same degree as adults. This is because of the upward movement of their growing spines. However, if headaches, neck pain, back pain, hip pain, or shoulder pain is present, it could be an indicator of a mild case of scoliosis. The likelihood of scoliosis becoming painful increases dramatically once an individual has stopped growing, which is another reason to take the signs of mild scoliosis seriously and proactively.

A Family History of Scoliosis

Although idiopathic scoliosis is *not* 100 percent caused by genetics, family members are often exposed to the same sets of factors and environmental conditions that can contribute to its development. Therefore, a family history of scoliosis could make it more likely that your child has a mild case.

When It All Adds Up

These signs of mild scoliosis, by themselves, may not indicate anything more than normal changes brought on by adolescence. But if two or more of these signs are observed, it may be time to consider seeing a professional to determine if the condition is, in fact, present. Again, the sooner scoliosis is diagnosed, the sooner proactive treatment can begin.

Understanding the Signs of Mild Scoliosis Can Lead to a Better Life

If you're concerned that your son or daughter may be living with mild scoliosis, a diagnosis marks a fork in the road on their journey through life. The traditional medical approach will recommend observation and inaction. But this only increases the possibility of worsening of the condition—and to a higher risk of possible expensive, invasive surgery.

Here at the Scoliosis Reduction Center, we understand the signs of mild scoliosis. Our team works with patients of all severity levels. In most cases, we're able to halt the progress of the condition completely, which allows patients to live their best possible lives.

Moderate Scoliosis—Facing Treatment Options at a Critical Time

When an individual's Cobb angle measures between twenty-five and forty degrees, experts classify the condition as moderate scoliosis. Although people with moderate scoliosis make up the majority of patients, this severity level remains something of a gray area for patients, parents, and even medical professionals. At this stage, the condition has progressed beyond mild levels and symptoms become quite obvious. But traditional approaches remain unconcerned with proactive measures for treatment, even when treatment would be highly beneficial.

Typically, individuals with moderate scoliosis would be diagnosed in adolescence. It's possible that they would have been diagnosed while the condition was still mild, but a large number of cases aren't caught until they reach the moderate stage. The reality at this point is that the abnormal spinal curvature is almost guaranteed to continue its progression when it reaches the moderate level. The progression may not happen rapidly, but it will happen.

Those with moderate scoliosis are usually told to continue watching and waiting until the condition becomes severe. Members of the medical establishment will claim that they simply don't know what might happen with the condition, despite overwhelming evidence indicating that moderate scoliosis progresses into severe territory more often than not. To me, this is a critical time for treatment, even if this period is a gray area. In my view, being proactive with treatment can help patients and family members avoid hardships down the road.

Time to Consider Bracing

Patients who have moved from mild to moderate scoliosis may be prescribed with a squeezing type of brace. The idea is that the brace will stabilize the spine and prevent its abnormal curvature from progressing further. Some research says that for adolescent patients, wearing a brace for at least thirteen hours each day can contribute to "successful" outcomes, meaning that curvatures don't progress to the stage at which surgery is necessary. But it will never reverse curvatures. Furthermore, teens who wear scoliosis braces such as the Boston or Milwaukee Brace exactly as prescribed can still experience a worsening of the condition. Other research indicates that bracing is simply ineffective. Why two conclusions from the research? Because a brace is only as good as the designer and fitter. Here at the Scoliosis Reduction Center, we use braces designed with correction and reduction—not just squeezing and holding—in mind.

Another factor to consider, as it applies to bracing, is the fact that it tends to take a massive effort on the part of parents and doctors to convince an adolescent patient to wear a cumbersome traditional scoliosis brace for the majority of their days. Teens are self-conscious, awkward, and sensitive enough as it is. Conventional bracing can actually produce a net negative effect. It may or may not stabilize an abnormal spinal curvature, but it will definitely impact a teen's life, socially and emotionally. And this impact can happen in ways that leave a lasting negative imprint.

The difference with the braces we use at the Scoliosis Reduction Center is profound because they're designed to be corrective. Patients experience actual improvements, which inspires them to become even more devoted to wearing the brace. Patients in our nontraditional braces feel more confident and in control because they don't see their scoliosis progress—they experience it improving.

The Signs of Moderate Scoliosis Are Easier to See

Moderate scoliosis usually produces some telltale signs and symptoms:

- The rotation and abnormal curvature of the spine is easier to notice with the naked eye.
- The position of ribs and/or shoulder blades becomes visibly more noticeable, particularly when a patient bends forward.
- Shoulders may take on an asymmetrical appearance.
- Overall, the body may become less symmetrical, causing posture to suffer.

For teens with scoliosis, these signs and symptoms signal changes that set them apart from their peers. And that's not a good thing! Traditional treatment approaches seem to ignore the emotional, psychological, and social impacts of the condition, always reverting to the mantra of "watch and wait." Of course, bracing is often prescribed at this time, but with traditional bracing designs, it is little more than a measure designed to delay the inevitable progression into severe territory, which is where surgery tends to be recommended.

The Chiropractic-Centered Approach to Treating Moderate Scoliosis Is Different

When patients with moderate scoliosis come to see me and my team at the Scoliosis Reduction Center, they experience a different reaction than they typically get when they encounter traditionally focused medical professionals. Instead of telling them to continue to watch and wait, we encourage them to take action. We also listen as they describe the ways in which the condition impacts their lives in ways that aren't physical.

We recognize our patients as complete human beings, and we understand that scoliosis is more than just a condition of the spine. When it has reached the moderate level of severity, it alters appearance and makes an individual's adolescence even more challenging than it would be otherwise.

I've noticed that this proactive approach gives patients confidence and a feeling of control over their condition. This helps to build self-esteem, and it gives teens reasons to feel good about themselves and their individual journeys. Our approach may be different, but the results our patients have experienced speak for themselves.

One key factor to keep in mind when it comes to treating moderate scoliosis is that there are major differences between traditional chiropractors and scoliosis-specific chiropractors. Treating scoliosis effectively with the chiropractic model requires special training and skills (outside of chiropractic adjustment) that traditional chiropractors are unlikely to possess. And as I mentioned previously in this book, there's a big difference between treating someone with scoliosis versus treating someone's scoliosis. Any chiropractor can treat someone with scoliosis by providing adjustments and general care. However, it takes a trained chiropractor to treat a person's scoliosis in a manner that effectively achieves a reduction.

Yes, there's great promise in treating moderate scoliosis with chiropractic care being the center of a holistic approach. However, the chiropractor needs to have a focus on scoliosis for it to have the desired impact. Otherwise, the condition could worsen.

Severe Scoliosis: Is It Too Late for Treatment?

Each case of scoliosis is as unique as the individual who has the condition. It affects different people in different ways, and there are varying levels of severity. Because the reality of dealing with scoliosis is different for each patient, treatment needs to be based on the particular needs of the individual and the severity of the condition. There simply is no one-size-fits-all treatment for scoliosis.

When it comes to severe scoliosis, however, traditional treatment methods almost always recommend surgery. Severe scoliosis comes with a high probability of the condition worsening. In fact, severe scoliosis carries a 90 percent risk of progression. That's why orthopedic doctors and others who treat the condition in the traditional manner recommend surgery. And it's why the condition needs to be taken very seriously.

If you or your child are dealing with severe scoliosis, you may feel pressured to opt for expensive and invasive surgery. Or you may assume that treatment options involving less invasive techniques aren't worth your time. But the truth is that there are effective options outside of surgery for those with severe scoliosis.

The Different Degrees of Scoliosis

As you have read previously in this book, traditional treatment methods recommend watching and waiting for mild scoliosis, with some doctors recommending exercises for their patients. Typical treatment guidelines recommend bracing, which only *attempts* to stop a progression, for those with moderate scoliosis. And, of course, surgery is often outlined as the only viable treatment option for those who have a severe case of the condition.

In reality, as scoliosis progresses, the traditional approach to treating it funnels patients to surgical solutions, regardless of the severity of the condition.

The watching-and-waiting approach usually leads to a progression and worsening of the condition. Inevitably, the scoliosis moves into the moderate or severe classification. If traditional braces are prescribed and used, they may slow the progression of the curve, but sooner or later, patients may find themselves at a point where surgery is recommended as the sole option for treatment.

I don't think it has to be this way!

I believe that proactive, chiropractic-centered treatment options can be implemented for patients, even the majority of those who have severe scoliosis.

Life with Severe Scoliosis

Once a case of scoliosis has become severe, it's important to know that surgery does not always prevent the continued progression of one's abnormal spinal curvature. The patient's Cobb angle can continue to increase even after the individual's spine has stopped growing. When scoliosis is severe, traditional bracing is also ineffective because the design of traditional bracing is meant to only hold a curve from progression. That's why surgery is so often recommended by surgeons.

Severe scoliosis also makes life more complicated for patients. It can contribute to daily, chronic pain, and it can place limits on a patient's lifestyle. Additionally, patients who live with severe scoliosis tend to be quite conscious of their posture, gait, and the way their clothes fit them. This makes them particularly sensitive to how others may treat them. Those with severe scoliosis also must deal with a heightened emotional component to the condition. Patients at this level may be more prone to experiencing a negative self-image, depression, substance abuse, or even suicidal thoughts.

Life with severe scoliosis can be challenging, to say the least. And when patients are faced with choosing invasive, expensive surgery as their only way forward, it can make them feel helpless.

A Different Way to Treat Severe Scoliosis

If you have severe scoliosis, is it too late for nonsurgical treatment? While surgeons may recommend surgery as the only relevant treatment option, I want patients and their families to know that alternatives exist.

When scoliosis becomes severe, treatment can be challenging for the patient. It requires a strong commitment, and results will not reveal themselves overnight. But I believe the difficulties faced by patients who choose less invasive treatment options pale in comparison to those who opt for surgery.

Numerous studies have highlighted poor outcomes for those who have been treated with surgery. And in many cases, a second surgery becomes necessary to remove hardware once the bone fusion has taken place. Surgery isn't guaranteed to reduce pain, disfigurement, or disability, either.

Here at the Scoliosis Reduction Center, our patients with severe scoliosis amaze me with their hard work and commitment to improvement. Together, we treat the condition using custom plans designed for each individual patient. Through chiropractic care, exercise, rehabilitation, and specialized, custom 3-D bracing, patients can avoid surgery and make significant improvements in their ability to get the most out of life. And if, for some reason, the nonsurgical treatments don't work, patients can always choose surgery at a later date. I just want to make sure that patients and their families understand surgery isn't their *only* option!

If you or your child are dealing with a case of severe scoliosis, you need to understand that not all roads lead to surgery! There are effective, alternative treatment options available. Yes, treatment will take time and effort, but it can help you find relief in a manner that's less invasive, less expensive, and more personally empowering than surgery.

Are You Experiencing These Seven Scoliosis Symptoms?

Life with scoliosis means living with a certain set of symptoms. Not everyone with scoliosis experiences the exact same symptoms. But some are so common and well-known that they're seen as signifiers of either the presence of the condition or the reality that the condition is getting worse.

Scoliosis symptoms can be obvious and not so obvious, which is why so many people live with the condition but go undiagnosed for such a long time. The fact is that people don't always know what to look for.

If you're concerned that you or someone you care about may have scoliosis, here are seven scoliosis symptoms you should be aware of:

#1—Changes in Posture or Body Symmetry

If you're concerned that your teenager or young child may have scoliosis, this is the symptom that will appear most evident. When an individual is affected by scoliosis, the appearance of the back, shoulders and hips may be asymmetrical or off center. Certainly, it is normal for a teenager to appear awkward during this stage of life—we're all familiar with the classic "adolescent slouch"—but there are some key indicators that you can look for:

- clothing hanging unevenly on the body
- one arm may seem to be longer than the other
- one hip may appear higher than the other
- one leg may appear longer than the other
- ribs or shoulder blades may stick out more prominently on one side of the body than the other

- arms held closely to the sides—with the waist or shoulders appearing unbalanced—instead of swinging naturally back and forth

#2—Impairments in Lung Function

Pulmonary function, which is a measure of how well the lungs perform, can be impacted negatively by scoliosis. The greater the curvature of the spine, the greater the impact on the lungs' ability to move air. The impact is most notable during exercise or other physical activity, but may be present during times of rest, as well.

#3—Neck, Back, Head, or Leg Pain

Because scoliosis affects the spine, it can have a negative impact on the body's nervous system, leading to pain and discomfort. Chronic, persistent pain in the neck, back, or legs may be caused by scoliosis. Muscle tension and frequent headaches may also be associated with scoliosis.

#4—Trouble Sleeping

Scoliosis can cause a chain reaction. The excess curvature of the spine can lead to pain and impairment in lung function, which in turn can impact one's ability to get a good night's sleep.

#5—Digestion Issues

It may be a difficult and odd concept to grasp, but scoliosis symptoms can include problems with digestion. Again, the spine is connected in some way to virtually every other body system, and curvature can affect the digestive tract just as much as it affects the muscles more closely connected to the spine. This can lead to difficulty with digestion and an inability to experience proper bowel function.

#6—Irregular Menstrual Cycles

The nerves that run through the spine connect the brain with all other organs, which is why sleep, digestion, and overall comfort are affected by scoliosis. Even menstrual cycles can become disrupted due to the condition and its impact on the body.

#7—Balance and Equilibrium Issues

Most people are adept at maintaining bodily balance with their eyes closed, and they're able to easily recognize their body position. The ability of the body to recognize its own position in the absence of visual cues is known as proprioception, and it's affected adversely by scoliosis, as is the ability to balance and maintain equilibrium. Balance and coordination can suffer as a result of scoliosis.

While most people are able to stand on one leg with their eyes closed for thirty seconds or more, people with scoliosis find this task quite difficult. An inability to do so does not necessarily mean that you have scoliosis, but it is a symptom that should be explored and evaluated.

Treating Scoliosis, Not the Scoliosis Symptoms

The symptoms I discussed above can be treated on their own, which may or may not lead to any lasting, significant relief. You can take aspirin for a headache or muscle pain, for example, but if your pain and discomfort is caused by scoliosis, no amount of any kind of pain reliever will address the root cause. Unfortunately, most approaches to health care in our society focus on the symptoms and not the underlying causes. This is why so many people suffer endlessly with chronic pain, discomfort, and an inability to participate in life to the extent that they would like.

Here at the Scoliosis Reduction Center, we believe that the only way to truly treat symptoms effectively is to address their causes. That is why we take such a comprehensive, proactive approach.

And the results speak for themselves. Most of our patients experience relief in a matter of just a couple weeks if they follow our procedures and do their homework!

Are you experiencing one or more of the symptoms mentioned here? Are you concerned that a scoliosis diagnosis may require you to cope with these symptoms for the rest of your life? We want to help! By addressing the causes of these symptoms, it's possible to improve your spine's strength and functionality considerably.

Scoliosis Can't Slow Down the World's Fastest Human

Members of the medical establishment talk a lot about the limitations of living with scoliosis. And because I want to discuss the condition comprehensively, it's necessary for me to shed light on those limitations as well. The difference with me is that I see those limitations as challenges that, when faced head on, can actually lead to breakthrough moments of positivity and the building blocks of remarkable personal character.

Scoliosis can be challenging to live with, but it does not have to prevent a patient from pursuing their passions. Just look at what the world's fastest human, Usain Bolt, has done with his life!

Usain Bolt is a remarkable individual: He is an eight-time Olympic gold medal winner and the holder of world records in the hundred-meter dash, the two-hundred-meter dash, and the four-by-one-hundred meters relay. He is the fastest, most decorated sprinter in history and a living athletic legend.

But what's most remarkable about Usain Bolt is the fact that he's accomplished all of this with scoliosis.

That's right—the world's fastest human has a significant abnormal spinal curvature. But he has refused to let it slow him down.

What's Usain Bolt's Secret?

Certainly, Usain Bolt is a gifted athlete with an amazing set of physical attributes. At a height of six five, he can use his long, powerful legs to take massive, nine-foot strides. You might think that because of his obvious talent and physical gifts, he would be even *faster* if he did not have scoliosis.

I have a different idea about what makes him special.

The world's finest athletes are physically gifted and talented, but the true superstars all share one thing in common—they're dedicated, hard workers. Usain Bolt has a tremendous work ethic, and he has applied his gritty dedication not only to running fast, but also to treating his scoliosis. The two things go hand in hand, in my opinion. Maybe Usain Bolt would be faster if he didn't have scoliosis. I think he's fast precisely *because* he has had to work so hard to overcome and treat his scoliosis.

This goes against conventional wisdom, obviously. But some of the leading experts in the biomechanics of sprinting suggest that Bolt's stride irregularities (his right leg strikes the ground with significantly more force than his left, and his left leg remains on the ground longer than his right) have actually forced him to optimize his abilities (New York Times, 2017).

Early in his career, Bolt experienced setbacks due to his scoliosis. He has said, "The early part of my career, when we didn't really know much about it (scoliosis), it really hampered me because I got injured every year." But then he and his training staff started looking into different types of treatment involving strength and conditioning exercises, as well as a more chiropractic-centered approach. Since then, Bolt says, "If I keep my core and back strong, the scoliosis doesn't really bother me. So I don't have to worry about it as long as I work hard."

Bolt uses an approach similar to the one we use here at the Scoliosis Reduction Center to treat his condition *and* enhance his performance. The combination of chiropractic techniques and sports rehabilitation practices—along with Bolt's willingness to put in the necessary hard work—is key to his ability to run faster than any human in history.

How Can You Be Like Bolt?

Living with scoliosis has traditionally meant that you would have to limit your life severely and hope that surgery might magically solve your condition. Usain Bolt's example proves this idea wrong. You may not have your sights set on Olympic gold medals or world records on the track, but you can draw inspiration from Bolt's approach.

The key, in my opinion, is to take a proactive—not reactive— approach to your condition. The traditional approach to scoliosis is a passive/reactive one that asks patients to wait and see what happens. I'm not saying that this approach should never be taken, but I think it's important to consider what's possible instead of dwelling on what's impossible because of scoliosis.

Usain Bolt has proven that scoliosis can be treated in a way that doesn't just reactively manage the condition. His example shows us that the spine can be strengthened and made more functional by using an approach like the one we take with our patients here at the Scoliosis Reduction Center. He also demonstrates that with hard work and dedication, just about any goal is attainable.

You can be like Bolt! But you will have to take charge of your condition and work hard. If you're like most of my patients, you have a lot of goals you want to achieve, and you aren't going to let scoliosis stand in your way. A fulfilling and functional life is possible through hard work and a proactive approach. You can change the course of your future, but it's only going to happen when you start considering what's possible instead of what's impossible.

Seven Reasons Why You Shouldn't Be Scared of Scoliosis

Whenever an individual receives a medical diagnosis, it's common for fears to arise. People wonder how certain conditions will affect their lives and relationships. They worry about their ability to participate in activities they love. And they feel anxiety about the unknown. This is particularly true when someone has been diagnosed with scoliosis.

Scoliosis fears are quite prevalent among those who have recently received their diagnoses, largely because the condition is so misunderstood. For parents, the worries are amplified because they fear the potential limitations on the lives and futures of their children. They want to ensure limitless possibilities for their young ones, but the threat of scoliosis limits those possibilities—or so they think.

I can understand exactly why scoliosis fears exist. As understood by the average person, scoliosis can only be treated effectively by undergoing expensive, invasive surgery. And because the condition is so misunderstood, misinformation dominates people's attempts to learn more, which only leads to greater fear and anxiety.

It breaks my heart to know that patients and parents experience such fear and anxiety surrounding scoliosis, especially when I know most of those fears are based on information that's untrue or outdated. Scoliosis is actually nothing to be afraid of.

I want to share my expertise so patients and parents can move forward proactively, confidently, and with a true understanding of the condition and its potential impacts. Armed with knowledge and awareness, people can make empowered decisions for treatment, taking steps that are no longer guided by fear.

Why Scoliosis Is Scary

The most common scoliosis fears are very persistent, but are mostly based on misunderstandings or untrue assumptions.

Generally, when patients and parents express their fears around scoliosis, they're concerned about surgery. Surgery is the mainstream standard of care for scoliosis, of course, so when a patient receives their diagnosis, their mind immediately goes to the operating room. They envision worst-case scenarios that involve outrageous expenses, extreme physical limitations, debilitating side effects, and the many potential dangers of surgery.

Young people with scoliosis aren't typically impacted by scoliosis pain, but they worry about how their condition will progress and how it will affect their lives in the future. They're often told that surgery is inevitable, which can be terrifying. While their peers plan for college and careers, young people with scoliosis find themselves preoccupied with fears about surgery and a highly limited adult life.

Some other common scoliosis fears include the following:

- possibility of severe deformity
- inability to become pregnant or carry a pregnancy to term
- life becoming characterized by increasing amounts of discomfort and pain
- reduction in the amount and types of physical activity that can be performed
- treatment that necessitates wearing a cumbersome, uncomfortable brace (that will not even reduce the curvature) most of the time
- making the condition worse by engaging in practices like carrying heavy objects or participating in sports
- collapse of the spine due to continuous progression

As much as I would like to tell patients and parents that they have nothing to fear, I respect that these fears are very real. However, I recognize that many of these very real fears are based on assumptions that aren't necessarily true.

People with scoliosis develop these fears because they have only been exposed to traditional, mainstream ideas about the condition and its treatment.

Thankfully, there are other, more promising perspectives on scoliosis.

Here are some of the reasons why a scoliosis diagnosis is nothing to be afraid of.

#1—Surgery Is Not the Only Treatment Method

Contrary to popular belief, surgery for scoliosis isn't inevitable. Taking a chiropractic-centered approach to treatment opens up a new range of possibilities, all of which are intended to provide relief and improvement *without* requiring surgery.

I believe that the mainstream approach to treatment is backward. Traditional treatment methods place people on the road toward surgery; instead, I believe that all treatment should be focused on *avoiding* surgery.

Here at the Scoliosis Reduction Center, we work with patients every day who once feared surgery. Thanks to our comprehensive, chiropractic-centered approach, they have been able to experience improvements without expensive, invasive operations. And with a continued focus on treating their condition through chiropractic care, therapy, exercise, and corrective bracing, they no longer need to feel dread about future surgery.

#2—Severe Deformity Is Extremely Rare

And it's even more rare when patients are proactive and undergo chiropractic-centered treatment. Watching and waiting, which is the traditional approach, can often lead to increased curvature and increased fear.

#3—Women with Scoliosis Have Normal Pregnancies and Births

Scoliosis does *not* cause any complications related to the ability to get pregnant, carry a pregnancy to term, or give birth. Additionally, it does not limit fertility, nor does it increase the possibility of miscarriage or birth defects. If you're a woman with scoliosis, or if you have a daughter with the condition, you can rest assured knowing that it will more than likely not have a negative impact on the ability to have children.

#4—People with Scoliosis Do Not Necessarily Need to Limit Physical Activity

Just look at Usain Bolt! By taking a proactive, chiropractic-centered approach, patients can live very active lives.

#5—Corrective Bracing Does Not Need to Be Cumbersome

Yes, traditional bracing apparatus are intimidating to young people with scoliosis, but there are alternatives. The ScoliBrace®, for example, pushes the spine into a corrected position, while the traditional bracing technologies squeeze the spine, causing discomfort.

#6—Scoliosis Is Not a Result of Carrying Heavy Objects

Many times, when a patient first receives their diagnosis, they wonder if it's their fault. Did they wear a backpack incorrectly? Did they lift too many heavy objects? Did they sit with improper posture? Will the scoliosis get worse by engaging in certain physical activities?

Scoliosis is *not* caused by wearing a backpack incorrectly or by lifting too many heavy objects. It is an idiopathic condition, which means that there's no single, known cause. Furthermore, patients can let go of fears about whether they will exacerbate the condition through their own actions. The truth is that the only thing that will increase the curvature of the spine is *inaction*.

#7—Spinal Collapse Is Highly Unlikely

Adults who fear a complete breakdown of the spine due to continuous progression of a curvature need not worry, especially if they take a proactive, chiropractic-centered approach to treatment.

Scoliosis Is Nothing to Be Afraid Of!

I understand why there are so many fears surrounding scoliosis, but I also know the truth about the condition. Yes, scoliosis can be scary. But when you're informed and you're willing to put in the work to treat the condition, you can live a normal, healthy, active life.

Life with Scoliosis Can Be Rich, Fulfilling, and Hopeful

The conventional wisdom about scoliosis has persisted for a long time. Decades, in fact. And because the traditional approach dominates the headlines regarding the condition, patients and parents see no reason to consider the condition as anything but a negative development.

As you can see, though, a narrative exists in which scoliosis isn't a life-altering hardship that only ends on the operating table. In fact, people are doing amazing things right now with curvatures that put them in the severe classification. And many patients are refusing to watch and wait until it's time for surgery or a spinal-fusion operation.

Life with scoliosis shouldn't be defined by anyone but the people living with it. I know firsthand that patients experience the condition in a multitude of different ways. I also know that there's reason to be hopeful with the condition. By working together, my patients and I can actually reduce curvatures, improve function, and do tremendous things in life with scoliosis!

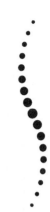

CHAPTER THREE

Scoliosis Advice, Wisdom, and Guidance

UNDERSTANDING THE NATURE OF scoliosis isn't something that can be taken for granted. There are many schools of thought and just as many ideas regarding appropriate treatment, which can make understanding the condition quite difficult. With so many voices weighing in on the subject, finding relevant advice and wisdom can seem impossible.

In chapter 1, I wrote about the facts surrounding scoliosis and what the condition actually *is*. In chapter 2, I discussed what life is like—and can be like—with scoliosis. Now I want to share some advice and wisdom that I know is helpful to scoliosis patients.

In my practice here at the Scoliosis Reduction Center, I see what works and what *doesn't* work in terms of dealing with the condition. But I also hear accounts of what it is like to be involved with the traditional approach to treatment, and I want to share what I know for patients and parents who only know the perspective supplied by the medical establishment.

I also want to share more facts and information to help parents of adolescents with scoliosis make better, more well-informed decisions. I believe that by educating people about scoliosis, we can live in a world where the condition doesn't cause so much confusion and stress.

Ask the Scoliosis Chiropractor!

For a variety of reasons, scoliosis is a condition that seems mysterious to many people—even those who have the condition themselves! It is fairly common among people of all ages, with more than four million people in the United States alone who have been diagnosed with scoliosis. And yet misinformation and misunderstandings of the condition persist.

As someone who deals with scoliosis on a daily basis, I get asked numerous questions about the condition fairly frequently. And I'm happy to educate, inform, and empower those who come to me seeking answers. To me, clearing up the confusion around scoliosis is an essential aspect of my job.

As a scoliosis chiropractor, I have a uniquely valuable perspective on the condition. It's a perspective that's been informed by a lifetime of interest, experience, and education. Most importantly, my knowledge of scoliosis grows every day thanks to my direct interactions with those who must live with the condition. They amaze me with their dedication to treatment and their passion for understanding scoliosis.

Why Understanding Scoliosis Matters

I decided more than a decade ago that I would use my expertise, talent, and knowledge to focus solely on scoliosis. I saw patients in my chiropractic practice who were scared, confused, and frustrated, and I knew I could do more to help them. I was also becoming increasingly frustrated by the conventional wisdom surrounding scoliosis.

These days I work almost exclusively with scoliosis patients. When I'm not practicing as a scoliosis chiropractor, I can be found speaking to others about the condition. This has taken me around the world, and it has introduced me to a wide spectrum of patients. What's more, every single member of my staff here at the Scoliosis Reduction Center is someone who has personally experienced the condition, has a family member with the condition, or has experienced relief from chiropractic-centered treatment.

There's a clear and undeniable correlation between an accurate understanding of scoliosis and a patient's ability to make proactive, healthy choices. The more patients and their families know, the more they can feel empowered to treat the condition effectively. They don't need to feel scared about inevitable surgery, and they don't need to live in confusion as they watch and wait.

In my interactions with patients and their families as a scoliosis chiropractor, I hear many of the same questions repeated. In the interest of helping as many people as possible, I thought I'd highlight some of those questions here, providing answers that readers can trust.

Let's get started!

Q: I have scoliosis. Does that mean my child will get it, too?
A: The quick answer is no. Most cases of scoliosis are idiopathic, which means that there's no single, known cause. Also, we know that scoliosis isn't hereditary. Yes, there may be genetic predispositions, but that does not guarantee that a member of a family will develop the condition.

That being said, parents who have scoliosis can be proactive by keeping an eye on their children and watching out for scoliosis symptoms. Although it's not hereditary, family members are often exposed to the same conditions that may contribute to scoliosis. The earlier it's detected, the simpler and more effective chiropractic-centered treatment will be.

Some of the early signs to look for include the following:

- uneven posture
- one leg seems to be longer than the other
- clothes fitting awkwardly
- presence of a rib hump
- head appears to be off center compared to the rest of the body
- spinal curvature visible to the naked eye

The bottom line is this: if you have scoliosis, it does not mean that your child will also develop the condition. However, being proactive and aware will help you create the best-case scenario for treating your child's scoliosis, should they develop the condition.

Q: What's the Cobb angle?
A: The Cobb angle is the most widely recognized measurement of a scoliosis curvature. Usually, it is measured by looking at an X-ray, which means that it is a measure of two-dimensional space. This means that the measurement is limited, since scoliosis is a three-dimensional condition. Conventional doctors who don't specialize in scoliosis may be able to tell that an abnormal curvature exists, but they don't have the expertise to measure a curvature accurately by looking at a single X-ray. That's why the Cobb angle measurement, by itself, can lead to a flawed understanding of the condition.

As a scoliosis chiropractor, I use multiple X-rays from numerous angles, not only to measure the true Cobb angle, but also to gain an accurate sense of the curvature in three dimensions. Scoliosis is treated most effectively as a three-dimensional condition; that's why we make sure we assess it three dimensionally, too.

Q: Is scoliosis surgery inevitable?
A: No. Although observation and surgery are the conventional methods of treatment, patients should understand that surgery doesn't have to be inevitable. In my opinion, surgery should only be seen as a last resort for patients who have tried chiropractic-centered treatments unsuccessfully, or those whose lives may be threatened without it. In my experience, abnormal curvatures can be treated effectively without surgery.

Q: Is bracing necessary to treat scoliosis?
A: It depends. Scoliosis braces such as the Boston Brace or Providence nighttime brace are commonly prescribed to adolescent patients, but they're nominally effective. Patients who undergo the conventional treatment approach are still often placed on a path that leads to surgery.

Here at the Scoliosis Reduction Center, we use bracing technology for many of our patients, but it is always used in conjunction with chiropractic care, physical therapy, and exercise. The braces we use also operate differently than the conventional ones. Traditional braces squeeze the spine, limiting function. Our braces *push* the spine in a manner that allows for correction of a curvature. They're also easier to wear in addition to being more aesthetically appealing.

Q: Can I die from scoliosis?
A: It is extremely unlikely. Scoliosis doesn't present a threat to patients' lives unless the spine's curvature becomes so severe that

it threatens internal organs. This is extraordinarily rare, though. What may be more likely to threaten a patient's life is surgery.

Scoliosis can cause pain, discomfort, and emotional hardships, but patients and their families need not worry about it being life-threatening. With a chiropractic-centered approach to treatment, curvatures can be reduced, providing relief to the body and its internal organs. When we reduce curvatures, we also reduce the need for surgery in the future.

Managing Expectations with Scoliosis

One of the keys to treating any medical condition is managing expectations. Successful outcomes are much more likely when everyone is on the same page. This means not only the patient, but also family members, loved ones, and members of the treatment team.

Unfortunately, expectation gaps emerge more often than not when so many different people become involved in the treatment of a condition.

What do I mean by that?

Let's say an adolescent patient has received a diagnosis of scoliosis. Typically, a parent will spend many hours researching the condition and developing expectations about the possibility of recovery. They will read about the traditional, surgically focused approach to treatment, but they will also spend some time looking at alternative treatments, some of which may be valid, while others are not.

Through this research, they will develop expectations. They may be overly skeptical and assume that surgery is inevitable, and that alternative treatment methods aren't worth pursuing. Or they may be overly optimistic and expect that their child will miraculously recover and resume normal activity within a very brief time frame. Because there's so much information to wade through, particularly online, the range of possible expectations is very wide!

Meanwhile, the adolescent patient is hearing anecdotal accounts from their peers about older siblings with the condition, or they're talking to classmates who live with scoliosis. They may even perform their own research into the condition. Along the way, they will develop expectations of their own. However, where the parent is likely looking at the condition from a longer-term perspective, the adolescent patient may be more focused on how the condition will impact their social standing in the here and now. Or they will focus on their ability to participate in activities they love.

At the same time, medical professionals are developing their own expectations based on their specific training, observations from viewing X-rays, analyzing the patient's medical history, and creating their own assessments. Under the traditional treatment model, a number of specialists may become involved in the care of the patient, which only multiplies the number of different expectations that are involved.

Additionally, friends, family members, and others bring their own expectations to the table—and almost no one is on the same page!

This is just one possible example; expectation gaps emerge all the time when dealing with scoliosis. But I don't think it has to be this way.

The Power of Open Communication
Expectations can't be managed effectively in silence. Communication is the key to ensuring success, regardless of the treatment path that's taken.

In my practice, I regard the setting and managing of expectations as a serious responsibility. After all, scoliosis is my main focus, so it is my duty to ensure that patients, parents, and loved ones understand the condition.

Here are some of the factors I discuss with patients and parents to ensure that we're all on the same page:

- **What is scoliosis?** I can't simply assume that everyone knows what scoliosis is, so I describe the condition as plainly and clearly as possible. This explanation establishes a baseline of understanding.
- **How has the scoliosis progressed?** Once everyone understands what scoliosis *is*, it's important to understand exactly how it is impacting that particular patient. Scoliosis is a progressive condition; it seldom remains static. So, it's critical for me to communicate the level of progression and curvature that exists. I also tell patients and parents about the risk of further progression and the rate at which it is likely to occur.
- **What is the patient capable of now?** It is crucial to assess the strength and flexibility of the spine upon diagnosis. In order to treat scoliosis effectively, everyone involved needs to understand the reality of the condition as it affects the individual patient. Two patients could have identical curvatures, yet the appropriate treatment approach could differ significantly based on each patient's current capabilities, flexibility, and strength level.
- **What does treatment look like?** This is very important. When I develop a plan for treatment, I ensure that patients and parents understand what the course of recovery will look like. When everyone understands what's necessary for treatment, accountability is much

easier to maintain. As I describe the treatment plan, I communicate the *what*, but I also describe the *how* and *why* of treatment. There should be no mystery regarding the reasons for a particular treatment approach.

• **Do you have questions?** Some patients and parents have pages and pages of notes, concerns, and questions. Others only have one or two questions. Regardless, open communication is a two-way street. So once I've shared what I know, I open the floor to patients and parents to ask questions, raise concerns, or just tell me how they feel about moving forward.

What Can the Average Patient Expect?

Of course, I can't speak for doctors and other medical professionals who represent the traditional model of treatment. I can only speak for myself and the treatment approach that I believe in. But if a patient becomes interested in the chiropractic-centered, functional approach to treatment, I want them to know what can be reasonably expected.

Obviously, every patient is different, but generally speaking, this is what I want patients, parents and others to understand about my approach:

1. **I can't cure scoliosis.** My patients have achieved some amazing results, but my approach to treatment does not cure the condition. However, I'm capable of stabilizing the spine and reducing abnormal curvatures using the functional approach.

2. **My goal is to prevent scoliosis from worsening and reduce curves.** Being scoliosis-free isn't the goal of treatment. This isn't as dismaying as it may sound. Consider those who live rich, full lives with high blood pressure or

diabetes. They have not cured their conditions, but they have prevented them from getting worse. My patients also live rich, full, active lives. They see noticeable improvements that allow them to be their best selves with a minimum of lifestyle restrictions.

3. **Treatment takes time.** In most cases of scoliosis, the condition has been present in the body for several years. Achieving reductions in abnormal curvatures does not happen quickly, but it happens. It's also important for people to understand that adapting to reduced curvatures takes time as well. Patients need to learn how to live with their improving spinal curvatures. They also need to understand that the brain, muscles, and other parts of the body require adjustment. It can be a long and sometimes grueling process, but to me it is far more attractive than the realities of dealing with surgery.

What Are Your Scoliosis Expectations?

Knowing what to expect after a scoliosis diagnosis is important. It's even more important to ensure that you're on the same page with your doctor and other professionals who may be involved in treatment.

Because the Scoliosis Reduction Center provides a comprehensive treatment approach, it's easier for me to ensure that my patients and I are always aligned when it comes to expectations. We provide chiropractic care, of course, but we also guide patients through a process that includes physical therapy, custom bracing, and scoliosis-specific exercises. Our patients find it easy to manage expectations because they aren't traveling from specialist to specialist. They're also kept in the loop about the realities of their treatment. Lines of communication are always kept open!

Five Ways Friends and Family Can Help after a Scoliosis Diagnosis

Scoliosis is a condition that affects millions of people who have been diagnosed with it. But it also has a major impact on the friends and family members of each person who has received the diagnosis. Individuals who have scoliosis are fortunate to receive the support of loved ones, but unfortunately, those loved ones don't always know how to provide the best, most appropriate support.

I know from working with countless scoliosis patients that no one overcomes the condition without help and support from others. Treating scoliosis effectively requires hard work and commitment not only from the patient, but also from the network of supporters surrounding the patient. My team and I provide the fundamental aspects of effective treatment, but friends and family members provide the essential emotional support and love that's necessary to drive a patient through treatment successfully.

Sometimes friends and family members offer support with their hearts in the right place, but their actions or words may actually be detrimental. Because scoliosis isn't well understood by members of the general public, people aren't always sure of what to say or do. Obviously, we don't want to discourage people from supporting those with scoliosis. But it is important to ensure that a patient's team of supporters understands what's helpful and what's *not* helpful.

To help friends and family members understand how they can provide the best support possible, I've come up with five ideas for providing help in the healing process.

Let's take a look!

#1—Understand the Realities of Scoliosis

The first step in providing helpful support is education. The average individual has a perception of scoliosis that might not be accurate or up-to-date. They may not fully understand the treatment options that are available today. They might be basing their knowledge of the condition on misinformation or secondhand accounts of experiences with scoliosis.

I encourage friends and family members to read and research the condition with open minds. It is important to let go of assumptions about scoliosis and learn about what it really means to have it. For those who are interested in learning more about scoliosis, this book is a wonderful resource. Chapter 1, in particular, is a great place to begin.

#2—Know What to Say—and What Not to Say

This is critical.

The most well-intentioned words can have a negative impact on scoliosis patients. Education can help people understand the realities of the condition, which can improve their ability to communicate about it respectfully. But it is also helpful to know some of the basics about the language we use to talk about scoliosis.

First of all, friends and family members should understand that people with scoliosis live rich, full, and active lives. They're normal people, just like anyone else. Therefore, they should be communicated with like normal people. They don't require people to be gentle with them in conversation. They just want to have normal, fun conversations like you or me!

Second of all, if a family member or friend is unsure of what to say, they should know that it is okay to ask questions. There's nothing wrong with displaying curiosity about the condition. Patients are usually happy to shed light on areas that are commonly misunderstood when it comes to scoliosis.

Finally, it can be helpful to know some of the things that friends and family members should *not* say to a scoliosis patient:

"I know someone with scoliosis, and..."
This is often said in an attempt to relate and empathize with the scoliosis patient, but it tends to backfire. Sometimes a person wants to tell the patient about a person they knew who turned out fine after receiving a scoliosis diagnosis. Or worse, they have negative stories to share about experiences people have had with scoliosis.

Every case of scoliosis is different, so it's not helpful to describe accounts of other people's experience with the condition. Instead, it's better to focus on the reality of the person who's experiencing the condition here and now.

"The curve looks fine to me!"
Often in an attempt to cheer up a person with scoliosis, a family member or friend will offer this assessment. I can understand why someone might feel like this is encouraging, but it's actually not helpful at all. Unless this assessment is coming from a doctor or a qualified scoliosis chiropractor, it's just not appropriate to say.

"You probably got scoliosis from..."
Once again, in an attempt to provide help and clarity to the scoliosis patient, a friend or family member may feel compelled to offer answers in the form of guesses as to how the condition started. They might mention other family members who have had scoliosis or make guesses about how certain activities contributed to the condition.

The truth is that most cases of scoliosis are idiopathic, which means that there's no known cause. Speculating about scoliosis causes is one of the least helpful things a person can do to provide support for the patient.

#3—Remember That the Patient Is More Than Their Scoliosis

Even though the condition can dominate their lives, scoliosis is just one aspect of the patient's existence. People with scoliosis come from all walks of life and have numerous interests. They're individuals with unique stories. Family members and friends should remember that scoliosis isn't the defining characteristic of the person they love.

#4—Practice Compassion

People close to a scoliosis patient can help just by taking time to consider what it must be like to live with the condition. This does not mean pitying or being condescending to the patient. Rather, it is about taking them at their word and showing understanding without attempting to solve the condition. The patient probably has the support they require on the medical front. What they need from their family members and friends is compassion.

#5—Accept the Patient for Who They Are

I work with all kinds of people who have scoliosis, and I'm lucky to get to know my patients as individuals. I don't see them as broken, and neither should loved ones. Scoliosis is a challenge to be faced, not a condition that defines an individual. Family members and friends can provide the best possible support simply by accepting their loved one as is.

Is Scoliosis Pain Keeping You from What You Love?

The experience of physical pain has a profoundly negative impact on a person's quality of life. When an individual feels pain, everything else recedes to the background, and life becomes focused exclusively on how to manage and/or eliminate the pain.

For people who have scoliosis, dealing with pain is particularly tricky. There are no quick fixes. And expensive, invasive surgeries are never guaranteed to diminish pain levels. Scoliosis pain affects lives negatively and keeps people from participating in the activities they love and enjoy. But for the average person dealing with the condition, there's no obvious solution when it comes to finding relief.

Making matters even more complicated, scoliosis pain doesn't typically make itself known until well into adulthood. And many people continue to subscribe to the myth that abnormal spinal curvatures don't contribute to physical pain. With so much confusion surrounding scoliosis pain, it's easy to understand why people resign themselves to lives of dealing with the condition using Band-Aid, stopgap solutions or by having surgery.

Are you being kept from what you love because of scoliosis back pain? Have you been told that the only way to find relief is through surgery? Are you worried that your pain levels will increase to debilitating levels as you age?

Thankfully, solutions exist to the problem of scoliosis pain!

Why Does Scoliosis Pain Increase with Age?

I want to tell you about the effective solutions that are available for people like you who deal with scoliosis pain on a consistent basis. But first, I want to address something that confuses a lot of patients.

If you have been dealing with scoliosis since you were a child, you may be wondering why pain has increased considerably in your adulthood. This is actually quite common. Adolescents with scoliosis rarely complain about pain; for them and their parents, the condition's negative aspects manifest as a decrease in function or an undesirable appearance. Pain is actually nonexistent or minimal for younger patients, and they're able to manage relatively full, active lives.

Once the body stops growing, however, scoliosis pain begins to present itself more aggressively. Why does this happen? In adolescence, the spine is continuously lengthening as the body grows. But when growth stops, the lengthening turns into compression, which places pressure on the spine and the surrounding nerves and tissue, which leads to pain. As the individual continues to age while leaving the condition untreated, the compression increases, which, in turn, increases the levels of pain.

Furthermore, adults are more likely to experience pinched nerves from degenerative scoliosis, which doesn't typically affect patients until they have reached the age of forty (CLEAR Institute, 2016).

The Scoliosis Pain Myth

Another confusing aspect of scoliosis pain is the persistent myth that it isn't real. If you're a person with scoliosis-related back pain, this probably seems outrageous to you! To you, it's obvious that your condition contributes to the pain you experience, and yet the myth about scoliosis back pain continues to linger.

It's true that spinal curvatures aren't inherently painful. But to suggest that they don't lead to real physical pain is silly. The areas of the body that surround the curve must adapt and contort in a manner that contributes directly to discomfort and pain, regardless of the severity of scoliosis. Again, this becomes exacerbated over time—adults join the workforce and must often endure long periods of standing or sitting. And as people get older, they tend to reduce the amount of healthy physical activity that's present in their lives, which contributes to ever-increasing levels of scoliosis pain.

Scoliosis pain doesn't just show up in the back, either. Many patients experience tension headaches related to abnormal curvatures in the upper-back area. These headaches can be especially exhausting, and can sometimes reach migraine-like levels of agony. What's more, scoliosis may lead to a decreased flow of cerebrospinal fluid (CSF), which can contribute to extraordinarily painful headaches.

In spite of the persistent myths about the condition, scoliosis pain is real! Fortunately, you don't have to believe the myths, and you don't have to settle for treatments that may or may not offer any relief.

Solutions for Scoliosis Pain

Thanks to a greater understanding of the condition and remarkable outcomes achieved through the chiropractic-centered approach to treatment, we now know that certain activities can help relieve pain and restore function for those with scoliosis.

- **Exercise**—Moving the body is incredibly beneficial for those with scoliosis. Bodies that experience motion regularly are more flexible and adaptable. They also have stronger muscles and more robust musculoskeletal systems, in general. Low-impact exercises like swimming, dancing, yoga, or road biking can have the effect of reducing pain. This is because they allow the body to better adapt to spinal curvatures. Of course, no exercise regimen should be attempted without first consulting a doctor!
- **Stretching**—Spinal curvatures lead to tightness, which leads to physical pain. This is because muscles on one side of a patient's body tighten in order to compensate for the curvature. Stretching can reduce tightness and help the

compensating muscles to relax, which can relieve scoliosis pain considerably.

- **Chiropractic-Centered Treatment**—Surgery is far from the best option for treating scoliosis pain. It is expensive and invasive, and can actually lead to increased pain and complications. The chiropractic-centered approach to scoliosis actually increases function, and it reduces pain as a result. This is the approach I use to treat my patients, and the results are nothing short of remarkable. I also help my patients with exercise, stretching, and the application of the latest techniques designed to reduce pain, improve function, and even reduce spinal curvatures!

You Don't Have to Live with Scoliosis Pain!

Understanding scoliosis is difficult because it impacts the body in so many ways. And persistent myths only add to the confusion. The truth is that you don't have to live with scoliosis pain! By taking the right approach, you can transform your body and your life, and you can get back to living the way you want while doing the things you love.

Scoliosis Side Effects: What You Need to Know

If you're exploring treatment options for any kind of medical condition, it's natural to be concerned about the associated side effects. And if you or your child requires treatment for scoliosis, you may be wondering if the effects of treatment are worth the relief that may be experienced.

The traditional scoliosis treatment approach typically leads to expensive and invasive surgery, so it's completely reasonable for you to be concerned. However, you should also know that the traditional approach isn't the only method of treatment that's available.

The chiropractic-centered approach to scoliosis treatment offers an alternative that I believe is far superior to the traditional approach. It is possible to reduce curvatures and improve function without having surgery. But you should understand that side effects are involved regardless of the approach you take to treatment.

Before you make any treatment decisions, I want to share some facts about scoliosis side effects, whether you're considering the traditional, surgical approach or not.

Let's get started!

The Side Effects of Scoliosis Itself

Before I get into the various side effects associated with different types of scoliosis treatment, I think it's a good idea to cover some of the consequences of doing nothing.

Scoliosis is an abnormal curvature of the spine, but it's also much more than that. The abnormal curvature affects the body and mind in a number of ways that you may not have considered.

Scoliosis and Pain

In many cases, scoliosis does not lead to physical pain. But the longer a patient lives with the condition, the more likely it is that they will begin to experience pain.

Pain from scoliosis can manifest in several different ways and in several different areas of the body. Left untreated, scoliosis side effects can include the following:

- headaches
- radicular (nerve) pain
- neck pain

- back pain
- hip pain
- knee pain
- leg pain

For the most part, scoliosis pain is experienced mainly by adult patients. However, roughly 20 percent of adolescents with the condition also experience muscle pain to some degree. And it only gets worse over time.

The Social and Emotional Components of Life with Scoliosis

Some of the more troubling scoliosis side effects aren't physical in nature. Instead, they manifest in a patient's social and emotional lives.

The abnormal curvature of the spine can create physical limitations that lead to social difficulties, especially for adolescents who may not be able to participate in certain activities with their peers.

Scoliosis can also affect sleep negatively, which leads to lower energy levels, irritability, and decreased performance in school or at work.

Maintaining a positive, optimistic view of life becomes more difficult when a person must deal with these side effects. Emotionally, people with scoliosis often must deal with anxiety or depression, which can be just as—if not more—debilitating than the physical side effects.

Other Scoliosis Side Effects

Leaving scoliosis untreated can lead to some other negative side effects:

- digestion issues
- negative impact on posture

- issues with balance and equilibrium
- an association with low bone density
- impacts on organ function (particularly in more severe cases)
- reduced oxygen intake

As you can see, scoliosis side effects can impact a patient in a variety of different ways. Certainly, treating scoliosis also comes with side effects, but the cost of doing nothing is too high to seriously consider such a passive approach.

The Side Effects of Scoliosis Surgery

Surgery is seen by many as the logical solution to the condition, and many patients go into surgery without an understanding of the impact it can have. In most surgeries for scoliosis, spinal discs are replaced with bone chips from the hip. Hooks, rods, and screws are also inserted into the body in order to keep the spine in place while it fuses. This is not a simple procedure, and the potential for experiencing negative side effects is high.

Some of the side effects of scoliosis surgery include the following:

- decreased flexibility and range of motion
- potential for further surgery if the spine fails to fuse properly
- wound infection
- potential for severe neurological deficits

If you're worried about these side effects, I can't blame you. Of course, surgeons do their very best to ensure positive outcomes for their patients, and the mortality rate for scoliosis surgery is very low. But surgery is complicated, highly invasive, and apt to lead to consequences that you probably have not considered.

The Side Effects of Scoliosis Bracing

Prior to surgery, the traditional approach to treatment usually involves the prescription of a scoliosis brace, such as the Boston Brace, Providence nighttime brace, or Milwaukee Brace. These devices must be worn for at least sixteen hours a day in most cases, and in some cases, they can be effective in terms of their ability to prevent scoliosis from getting worse. That being said, there are a number of associated physical, emotional, and psychological side effects that stem from being confined to such a brace for long periods of time:

- depressed mood
- physical limitations that can reduce one's overall quality of life
- increased stress
- a decrease in self-esteem
- decreased flexibility
- social isolation and anxiety
- negative body image
- pain and sores from the pressure the brace exerts on the body

While traditional scoliosis bracing has been shown to help prevent the progression of the condition in some studies, it comes with consequences that patients and parents may not be willing to endure.

Note that these are the side effects common to traditional bracing apparatus. The braces we use here at the Scoliosis Reduction Center are corrective, and operate much differently.

The Side Effects of Chiropractic-Centered Scoliosis Treatment

The type of treatment we provide here at the Scoliosis Reduction Center is chiropractic-centered. We don't take patients down a path that leads to surgery, and our scoliosis bracing technology works in a manner that does not lead to the side effects listed above. With this approach, patients can reduce their curvatures and improve flexibility and function. And the side effects are minimal.

Patients who come to us for treatment should be prepared to put forth an effort that can leave them feeling exhausted, but in a manner that's more like the feeling of a tough workout regimen. The treatment is multifaceted and intense, but our results speak for themselves!

Scoliosis: An Emotional Journey

Scoliosis is a condition of the spine, and it has significant effects on the human body. Therefore, most scoliosis experts discuss the condition in terms of the physical. But I think it's just as important to recognize its emotional impact. A full, comprehensive, and successful approach to treatment can't focus solely on the body and the abnormal spinal curvature; it must also focus on the emotional journey.

Whether a patient is an adolescent or an adult, scoliosis will have a considerable impact on emotions. Teens typically find themselves riding on an emotional roller coaster under normal circumstances. When scoliosis is also a part of the picture, it adds another emotional dimension that can be extremely difficult to deal with. Adults with scoliosis may be better suited to handle the emotions that come with the condition, but they still require support and understanding from others.

I want patients and their families to know that it is completely normal for scoliosis to have a profound impact on emotions. I can't cure a negative emotional state, nor can I prolong a positive one; emotions come and go. But I *can* help by offering my knowledge and wisdom and by maintaining an open dialogue. The most important thing is to ensure that patients are heard. They need to understand that their emotional challenges are valid and that they have a real impact on living life with scoliosis. I'm here to listen, but I also recognize the importance of relating to others what scoliosis patients experience on an emotional level.

Constant, Continuous Bad News

Scoliosis patients are rarely given reason to hope. In most cases, they're given bad news every single time they see a doctor or specialist. The reason for this is that scoliosis is a progressive condition that generally does not remain static. Even when a patient follows their doctor's orders precisely and wears a Boston Brace for twenty or more hours a day, the best they can hope for is the maintenance of the status quo.

Imagine having a medical condition that only worsened over time. Imagine being told bad news on a continuous basis. It would be quite difficult to maintain a positive, upbeat emotional state under those circumstances, wouldn't it?

The progressive nature of scoliosis does not allow for breaks in the constant flow of bad news. It does not typically allow for patients to feel like their proactive efforts are leading to improvements. And it does not allow patients to feel very hopeful.

This reality is particularly difficult for adolescents with scoliosis to endure. The teen years are notoriously difficult and awkward, but at least most teens get to experience normal ups and downs, with the highs offsetting the lows. Unfortunately, for teens with scoliosis, the condition plays a major role in nearly every aspect of life. There are few highs to offset the lows, and this wreaks havoc on an already unstable emotional landscape.

Physical and Emotional Relief: Traditional Treatment

Being exposed to continuous bad news about scoliosis takes a toll on emotions. However, the promise of relief can mitigate the negative emotional impact.

Patients who receive traditional treatment look forward to the promise of a surgical solution. This gives them hope and helps them imagine a life in which scoliosis isn't a primary concern. Sadly, the hope they feel isn't without negative consequences. Surgery is expensive, invasive, and risky. And it isn't guaranteed to improve the condition. It may produce a straighter spine, but with the serious consequences of spinal fusion. Nevertheless, it can provide physical relief, which often translates to emotional relief as well. Unfortunately, this relief may only be replaced by other issues over time. And these issues may even be worse, post-surgery, than they might have been without surgery.

Physical and Emotional Relief: Chiropractic-Centered Treatment

On the other hand, patients who receive functional, patient-centered treatments like those offered here at the Scoliosis Reduction Center can look forward to actual reductions in the severity of their spinal curvatures—without surgery.

Every day, each one of our patients makes progress on an emotional journey. At first, it is quite difficult. They're incredibly eager to experience relief, but they can be intimidated by the process. We ask a lot of our patients in terms of their ability to participate actively in their own recovery. It involves a lot of hard work, as well as some patience. Results don't become evident overnight.

Eventually, the collaborative work that our staff members perform with our patients begins to pay off. You can see the positive emotional changes written on their faces. As their spinal curvatures improve, they begin to notice welcome changes in appearance and function. Their clothes start to fit a little better. They become more flexible and functional, too, which boosts confidence and creates a positive emotional uprising. They begin to change their perspectives on the future, as well. Patients who once saw the future as bleak and scary start seeing the coming weeks, months, and years in a much more optimistic light.

After about ninety days, the anxiety that patients have become so accustomed to starts to fall away. They can tell that they're getting better and that their hard work is paying off. They engage in their treatments with greater enthusiasm, and they express gratitude for the changes they experience.

This emotional journey isn't the same for everyone. But for those who engage in chiropractic-centered treatment for scoliosis, it happens this way more often than not. And it makes me extraordinarily proud of the work my staff and I do.

Ultimately, helping people improve the emotional impact of scoliosis is just as important as helping them physically. The two aspects go hand in hand. In my opinion, you can't have one without the other!

Three Signs of Scoliosis for Concerned Parents

So far in this chapter, I've provided some answers and guidance for those who may be confused about scoliosis, or who may have bought into some misinformation regarding the condition. There's a lot that's not well understood about scoliosis, in general, especially when it comes to topics like side effects, emotional impacts, pain levels, and appropriate expectations.

My focus for the next few sections of this chapter is on parents of adolescents with scoliosis. They may or may not have the condition themselves; regardless, they often find themselves in the dark in terms of their understanding of the condition.

Parenting a child who has adolescent scoliosis can be almost as confusing and frustrating as being an adolescent! That is why I want to share my knowledge here with you.

If you're a parent, there's nothing more important to you than the health and well-being of your child. You feel every cough and sniffle with them, and you bear the pain of the occasional scraped knee or elbow just as much as they do. You treat your child with love, and you do everything in your power to ensure a safe, happy, and healthy future.

Unfortunately, some conditions aren't as easily noticed as a cold or a playground injury.

Scoliosis is the most common deformity of the spine in children, with literally millions of young people in the United States alone who have the condition. Nearly 30,000 scoliosis surgeries are performed each year on adolescents in the United States. It has a profound impact on the lives of children and adolescents, but it can be treated effectively and less invasively if you take a proactive approach.

The signs of scoliosis aren't always obvious, unfortunately. However, if you educate yourself on what to look for, you can put your child on the path to living their best possible life much sooner—and much more effectively!

Are you unsure of what to look for if you're concerned your child may have scoliosis? I've compiled a list of the signs you should be seeking. Let's take a look!

#1—Changes in Posture and Appearance

The most obvious, telltale signs of scoliosis in adolescents are related to posture, symmetry, and the appearance of the hips, shoulders, shoulder blades, and back. You may notice clothing hanging unevenly on your child, or you might realize that the distance between the arm and torso is greater on one side of the body than the other.

Other signs of scoliosis related to posture and appearance include the following:

- ribs protruding more on one side than the other
- ribs protrude while engaging in a full forward bend
- problems or unevenness during motion
- arms held tightly to the side while walking
- one hip more prominent than the other
- head not centered evenly over the body
- one shoulder or shoulder blade higher or more prominent than the other
- one leg appears shorter than the other
- pant legs, necklines, hemlines, and shirtsleeves appear uneven
- eye line appears to be tilted
- spinal curvature visible to the naked eye

These scoliosis signs are the most obvious, and they represent symptoms of the underlying cause.

#2—Difficulty Balancing

Balance and coordination are also affected by the presence of scoliosis in young people. This may not be as apparent as the signs mentioned above, but it can indicate that your child has the condition.

Often, people with scoliosis have problems with their ability to recognize the position of their own bodies. This ability, known as *proprioception,* can be diminished in people with scoliosis. Your child may not admit that they're having trouble with balance or coordination, but if you suspect possible issues, you can have them stand on one leg with their eyes closed for thirty seconds. If your child has difficulty remaining stable, it could be a sign of scoliosis.

#3—Tiredness and Fatigue

We all know that teens and other young people can never get enough sleep! But if your child seems excessively tired and fatigued much of the time, it could be because of scoliosis.

As spinal curvatures progress and become more pronounced, the muscles surrounding the spine are forced to exert more energy and work harder just to keep the body properly balanced and aligned. What's more, as scoliosis becomes more severe, pressure can be placed on the chest cavity, which can restrict breathing, leading to increased feelings of fatigue.

If your child is constantly complaining of being tired or worn out, even after exerting very little energy, it could be a sign of scoliosis.

You've Seen the Signs—Now What?

These signs and symptoms may be caused by scoliosis, or they may be a result of something else entirely. The only way to know for sure whether your child has scoliosis is to get them examined by a doctor, which will involve having X-rays taken.

Once a diagnosis has been made, experts may tell you that the best approach going forward is to watch, wait, and see what happens. But I know that for you and your child, that's simply not good enough!

Here at the Scoliosis Reduction Center, we believe in giving our young patients the best chance at a full, rich, and active life, and that means taking a proactive, chiropractic-centered approach. With the help of our team, your child does not have to be limited by scoliosis. Instead, they can continue growing, learning, and staying active with the rest of their peers.

Four Facts about Scoliosis Treatment for Teens

I bet it's not difficult for you to remember what your life was like between the ages of ten and eighteen. The adolescent years are a magical time for many of us, and if you're like me, the experiences you had as a teen helped to mold you into the person you are today. Sadly, many teens who have been diagnosed with scoliosis must adjust their lifestyles, choices, and plans for the future. Traditional scoliosis treatment options for teens also tend to negatively impact the ability to make the most of what should be a positive and memorable time.

What Is Adolescent Idiopathic Scoliosis?

Adolescent idiopathic scoliosis (AIS) is actually the most common form of the condition. Idiopathic means that there's no known cause, which is a fact that frustrates teens and their parents. Regardless of the cause, however, scoliosis treatment approaches should take into account the needs, preferences and future goals of the patient.

AIS affects 4–5 percent of adolescents, which may not seem like a large number, but it is significant. This is especially true when you consider the impact that such a condition has on the trajectory of a young person's life.

Symptoms include a rib hump, which is usually the most obvious, visible sign of the condition, asymmetrical shoulder heights, and torso lean, which is a shift of the body to either the right or left that creates the appearance of one hip being higher than the other.

Teens don't always experience pain in association with AIS, largely because of the upward, lengthening motion of the body's growth during this time. By contrast, adults with scoliosis tend to experience more pain because once they have stopped growing, the tendency is for the spine to compress, which leads to pressure that causes pain and discomfort.

Because pain is rarely expressed—or even evident—teens should be examined for abnormalities in their body symmetry and posture. Further examinations can reveal a curvature of the spine. If the curvature is greater than 10 degrees, the adolescent is diagnosed with scoliosis.

What Happens after Diagnosis?

Once a diagnosis has been made, parents and their adolescent children are faced with some critical decisions. Traditionally, a wait-and-see approach is taken with teenage patients. When spinal curves become severe, though, scoliosis treatment approaches such as surgery will be recommended. If the child is still growing and developing, grow rods may be implanted, which will require subsequent procedures as the child continues to grow. If the child is older and closer to the conclusion of their growth period, spinal-fusion surgery is recommended as a remedy for scoliosis.

If you're the parent of an adolescent who has been diagnosed with scoliosis, you probably have a lot of concerns and questions running through your mind.

- Will the curve continue to worsen?
- Will my son or daughter be able to participate in sports and other activities?

- Will scoliosis impact my daughter's ability to have children in the future?
- Will my teen require surgery, and if so, how will that affect their ability to participate in school?
- Will my son or daughter be forced to limit their potential career choices?
- Is surgery the only option when the curve becomes severe?
- Is there anything that can be done to avoid invasive surgery?

To help you better understand the impact that AIS will have on your child, here are some important scoliosis treatment facts for teens:

#1—You Don't Have to Just Watch and Wait

The traditional approach to adolescent scoliosis treatment suggests that while the body is still developing, very little can be done to improve functionality and reduce the curvature of the spine. Sadly, this approach almost always leads to expensive, invasive surgery, whether it's during your child's adolescence or at some point in adulthood. You don't have to wait it out, though. In fact, alternative treatment options allow your son or daughter to strengthen their spine while improving functionality and preventing additional curvature. This gives them a chance to participate fully in all the activities that are so crucial to their adolescent life.

#2—Scoliosis Treatment Does Not Need to Limit Your Child's Career Path or Future Family Plans

When surgery is the ultimate outcome of a treatment approach, it's easy to see why it might affect the ability to select a more active career path. But when alternative approaches are taken, anything is possible. For example, General Douglas MacArthur was initially refused entry into West Point Academy due to his scoliosis. But he engaged diligently in spinal exercises that improved his strength and mobility. Later, he was admitted to West Point, and the rest is history!

Additionally, in most nonsurgical cases, the ability to become pregnant and have healthy children isn't affected—even when large curves are present. In surgical cases, it will not affect the ability to have children, but it should be noted that the patient can experience more pain during pregnancy.

#3—Scoliosis Treatment Is Not Limited to Surgery

If you have been made to believe that surgery—along with the associated complications and costs—is inevitable, you will be pleased to know that alternatives exist. In fact, alternative treatments that employ a host of modalities including chiropractic care can give your teen an even richer and fuller life than the surgical path promises, at a fraction of the cost.

#4—Early Diagnosis Increases Scoliosis Treatment Options

Please don't wait to have your adolescent child screened for scoliosis! Checkups should happen regularly—at the very least, once per year. Your teenage son or daughter is unlikely to complain about discomfort or pain, so it's up to you to be proactive. And because adolescence is the timeframe when children become more private and independent, you need to be extra diligent about ensuring their good health. A scoliosis diagnosis may be difficult to hear, but when it happens sooner than later, it gives you and your child the chance to set foot on a path that makes them stronger and better able to live an unlimited life.

Do You Have More Questions about Scoliosis Treatment for Teens?

You love your child, and the last thing you want is for them to miss out on their adolescence because of scoliosis—or because of the necessity of scoliosis surgery. Whether your adolescent son or daughter has received a scoliosis diagnosis or you're simply concerned that they may have the condition, you probably have a lot of questions about what comes next. Fortunately, answers are available! This book contains the facts about scoliosis, but if there are lingering questions in your mind after reading, please feel free to reach out to us here at the Scoliosis Reduction Center!

How to Help Your Teen Deal with the Emotional Impact of Scoliosis

Scoliosis is a physical condition of the body, but its emotional impact shouldn't be underestimated. We talk a lot about the physical and medical aspects of scoliosis. The rate at which curves progress, the types of treatments that are most effective, and the limitations that must be dealt with are all topics deserving of discussion. But for many people, the emotional aspects of living with scoliosis have the greatest impact. This is especially true for adolescents with the condition.

Teens are incredibly emotional creatures to begin with. The dramas that play out in their day-to-day lives involve challenging interpersonal relationships, the pressures of school, and the many confusing changes that happen within their bodies. These are exciting times, but they're deeply emotional periods in the lives of people. And when a teen must also deal with a scoliosis diagnosis, emotions become even more complicated and difficult to deal with.

If you're the parent of a teen with scoliosis, you probably recognize that your child is riding on an emotional roller coaster. But you may not understand just how much their condition impacts the changing tides of emotion. Of course, you want to do your best to ensure that your adolescent son or daughter makes the most of their teen years. But what can you do when the emotional issues of adolescence are amplified by scoliosis?

To me, the first step to helping your child is to understand what they're going through.

Scoliosis and Adolescent Relationships

Teens crave meaningful connections with their peers. They yearn to belong and to be accepted. Scoliosis does not make this easy!

When a teen's posture is uneven, or their clothes don't quite fit properly, they can feel extremely self-conscious. Those who have been fitted with traditional, non-corrective, and bulky scoliosis braces are even more susceptible to challenging emotions associated with building and maintaining healthy relationships. Let's face it—kids with scoliosis stand out, and they feel it when the eyes of their peers are trained on them because of their condition.

Studies have shown that the majority of scoliosis patients struggle with relationships. Many of them become shy or begin to isolate themselves from others. Social situations can be emotional mine fields for teens, leading some to avoid socializing as a defense mechanism. According to research, teens with scoliosis spend less time dating and participating in recreational activities than their contemporaries who don't have the condition.

Struggles with Self-Esteem

Body-image issues, especially for girls, are common in the adolescent population. Having an abnormally curved spine only exacerbates such issues. As you know, teens can act cruel to one another, often focusing on exactly the areas that their targets feel most self-conscious about. This makes fitting in very difficult for adolescents with scoliosis. They can internalize the comments they hear and begin to feel unattractive and uncomfortable.

Teens with scoliosis are far more likely to feel ashamed of their bodies compared to their peers. More than half of them feel dissatisfaction with the way they appear. And there's a tendency for teens to obsess about body image. You may notice your child frowning as they view themselves in the mirror or talking disgustedly about their curves.

Mental Health and Emotional Well-Being

The issues I've outlined thus far are serious, but they can actually lead to even more significant, major problems if they aren't addressed.

The emotional impact of scoliosis on adolescents sometimes leads to long-term mental-health concerns like depression and anxiety. It's not uncommon for teens with scoliosis to report feeling empty inside. Consequently, adolescents who have scoliosis are more likely to consider suicide than their peers.

Teens who experience these types of emotional upheavals look to substances like alcohol and drugs for relief. Adolescents with scoliosis engage in substance abuse at rates far higher than their peers. For example, girls with scoliosis are three times more likely to consume alcohol than their peers who don't have scoliosis. And boys with scoliosis drink almost twice as much alcohol than their peers.

These emotional impacts should be taken very seriously. They represent more than just a phase that your child is going through. They can have long-term and far-reaching impacts on your child's entire life.

What Can Parents Do?

Being the parent of a teen is hard work. Being the parent of a teen with scoliosis is much more difficult. But it's also extraordinarily rewarding when you're able to guide your son or daughter successfully through their adolescence in spite of the impacts of their condition.

The most important thing you can do for your child is to establish and maintain open lines of communication. Don't just limit your discussions of scoliosis to the physical realities of the condition; encourage your child to talk about how their scoliosis makes them feel. Take time to ask questions. And make sure you truly listen to what they have to say. Simply giving your son or daughter the opportunity to express themselves openly and honestly will provide enormous relief.

When you speak with your child, it's critical that you communicate without judgment. Their emotional turmoil may seem trivial to you as an adult. But to them, there's nothing more consequential than the emotional matters they're dealing with right now.

Finally, I would encourage you to continue educating yourself about the condition and its impact on your adolescent child. Seeking information and support will show your son or daughter that you're in their corner and that their struggles mean something to you. The more you know, the more you will be able to provide help during a difficult time in your child's life.

Scoliosis and the Power of a Positive Mental Attitude

Scoliosis is obviously a physical condition of the spine. In most cases, it's assessed and treated in terms of its impact on the body, which makes perfect sense. However, scoliosis affects much more than just the body. It impacts emotions, mood, and other human characteristics in significant ways. In fact, I would argue that treating scoliosis is as much of a mental and emotional endeavor as it's a physical one.

As you read in the previous section, it's crucial for parents, patients, and others to understand the significant emotional impact scoliosis has on adolescents. A positive mental attitude is perhaps the most powerful tool available for facing the emotional challenges of the condition. Patients who approach treatment—and life in general—with positive mind-sets are much more likely to find success in treating their scoliosis. Parents who stay positive are more present and better able to provide meaningful support to their adolescent children with scoliosis. And adults who have the condition also experience considerable benefits from a mental attitude characterized by positivity.

Of course, a scoliosis diagnosis can make it quite challenging to establish and maintain a positive mental attitude. Adolescents hear horror stories of their peers who must spend most of their waking lives in cumbersome braces that only provide a small chance of preventing further progression. And they're often told that they must become accustomed to a life of limitations because of their condition. Adults who have scoliosis may not face the specific social pressures that teens must contend with, but it's no less difficult for them to stay positive, especially when you consider that traditional treatment options offer very little hope in terms of actually reducing curvatures.

We know that one's mental makeup affects treatment in significant ways. And we see the power of positivity every single day here at the Scoliosis Reduction Center. But how can patients, parents, and others cultivate positivity in the first place?

What Positivity Can Do for Scoliosis Patients

A positive mental attitude isn't just something that's nice to have when facing a condition like scoliosis. It actually helps in specific, measurable ways.

According to the Mayo Clinic, positive thinking comes with a number of potential health benefits:

- longer life span
- greater resistance to illnesses such as the common cold
- lower rates of mood disorders such as depression
- lower levels of negative stress
- improved cardiovascular health
- reduced risk of death from cardiovascular disease
- improved coping skills for stress and other hardships

While it's unclear exactly why these health benefits arise from a practice of positive thinking, we know that a positive mental attitude tends to be accompanied by a healthier response to stress.

Stress can be incredibly harmful to the physical body. Although it's experienced primarily as a mental or emotional challenge, stress creates real tension in the body's tissues. It also increases the production of cortisol, which is commonly known as the *stress hormone*. Cortisol, which has been described by Psychology Today as "Public Enemy No. 1," interferes with learning and memory (Psychology Today, 2013). It also decreases immune function, reduces bone density, leads to weight gain, heart disease, and more. Cortisol also increases an individual's risk of depression and contributes to lower life expectancy.

For the average person, this can make them more suscep-tible to a host of conditions. For a person with scoliosis, stress and its aftereffects can exacerbate the impacts of the condition and negatively impact a person's ability to heal effectively. These effects are amplified in adolescents, who are already on emotional high alert.

A positive mental attitude is the best defense against stress. But cultivating an attitude of positivity in the midst of dealing with a life-changing condition like scoliosis can seem impossible. Fortunately, for many patients and parents, simply becoming aware of the benefits of a positive mental attitude is enough to encourage them to consider the ways in which they can transition to a sunnier, more optimistic worldview.

It's important to note that developing a positive mental attitude isn't about avoiding negative feelings and emotions! Those are normal and expected. In fact, I would be alarmed if I ever encountered a completely cheerful patient. Staying positive does not mean glossing over negative emotions or pretending they don't exist. Instead, it's about a deliberate, intentional choice to see the bright side of situations, even in the face of negative aspects of one's condition.

An individual with a positive mental attitude doesn't ignore setbacks or gloss over undesirable aspects of their condition. Rather, they mindfully acknowledge reality and consider the fullness of life. Yes, there are some negative aspects of dealing with scoliosis. But they don't dwell on them or allow them to spiral out of control, leading to greater stress and strain. Instead, they face them head on. Then, they make a deliberate choice to move ahead with a positive mental attitude.

Sugarcoating the reality of scoliosis isn't what being positive is about. Scoliosis *is* a big deal, and it can lead to invasive surgery if it's treated improperly. Therefore, the sooner a patient understands the reality of the condition, the better. Scoliosis may be a big deal, but that doesn't mean it can't be handled with positivity in the midst of realism.

The Keys to Developing a Positive Mental Attitude

Cultivating positivity is a practice. It does not happen overnight. Patients, parents, and others must continually work at it. It's about developing habits that become ingrained in a person's day-to-day lifestyle. It takes time and a bit of effort, especially when it comes to restructuring well-established negative thought patterns. But it's something that definitely can be done.

Here are some of the best ways to develop a positive mental attitude in the face of scoliosis:

Exercise

Although it may seem counterintuitive, the most effective way to transform an emotional landscape defined by negativity is to engage the body physically. Exercise burns up the stress hormone cortisol and prevents it from manifesting in the many troubling ways I mentioned above. Physical activity also provides an outlet for the fight-or-flight response that so often accompanies stress. And of course, exercise impacts the body in a number of positive ways, which leads to improved self-esteem, higher energy levels, and a more positive response to treatments and therapies.

Scoliosis patients may be wary of participating in physical activities because they fear potential harmful impacts to their bodies. I understand this hesitation, but I encourage patients to participate in sports and other activities because they can actually strengthen the body and create better physical conditions for healing. Of course, everyone with scoliosis is different, so I recommend consulting with a doctor or scoliosis chiropractor before engaging in physical activity.

Meditation/Mindfulness

Scoliosis patients and the people who care for them experience a never-ending stream of thoughts and emotions that can vary wildly. Sometimes it can feel like too much, or that the emotional, mental rollercoaster is out of control. A mindfulness practice helps patients and others develop an awareness of their own thought patterns. When a person is aware of what's happening in their mind, they gain the power to change things. This is the power of mindfulness.

A regular meditation practice can help with the development of mindfulness, but the process need not be formal. In fact, just paying attention more to the present moment, regardless of what might be happening, is one of the most effective ways to cultivate a mindful presence. Again, this is all about developing new habits, which is why the practice needs to be done regularly.

Scoliosis patients who are aware of the thoughts and emotions they experience are better able to create mental space for positivity. Parents and others who develop mindfulness are more present for their loved ones and have a greater capacity to provide positive care.

Social Activity

Human beings are social animals. Regardless of whether a person is introverted or extroverted, spending time with other people is one of the surest ways to improve mood and heighten feelings of positivity. Isolation can be extremely harmful for people, particularly adolescents who may be feeling especially troubled by the effects of their condition in addition to the normal issues associated with teenage years.

The bonds people share with each other are powerful in the healing process, and they lead to a greater sense of positivity. Face-to-face time with others in real life is excellent medicine, but even interacting positively with others online or in other virtual spaces can have beneficial impacts.

Not all social settings are appropriate for developing a positive mental attitude, though. Parents and scoliosis patients should seek out groups of people who are positive, welcoming, and supportive. Spending time with negative-minded individuals can do more harm than good, so it's important to focus on the people who engage in interactions with warmth, love and hope. If a patient can find other individuals who have achieved success in treating scoliosis, those connections can be the most beneficial and meaningful.

Laughter

This goes hand in hand with social activity. Laughter lightens the mood and can make almost any situation seem less troubling. Watching sitcoms and comedy movies can help, but the best laughs are those that come from social settings with loved ones. Laughter eases tension in the body and helps to minimize negative thought patterns. It's also connected to a reduction of the stress hormone cortisol.

Getting Results

To me, the absolute best way to cultivate a positive attitude—and maintain it—is to achieve results through treatment. All the other methods of cultivating a positive attitude pale in comparison. Positivity is hard to come by when results aren't being achieved. However, when the correct treatment is applied and patients begin to see results, it has an incredible impact on the ability to stay positive.

I know this because I often see patients come into the clinic who have received—or are currently receiving—traditional treatment. Their moods and demeanors are almost uniformly negative, and their parents typically feel defeated, too, because treatments have not worked. Turning an attitude like this around can be difficult if someone has applied an honest effort, but it just didn't work. Thankfully, I've seen on numerous occasions that once patients and parents engage actively with chiropractic-centered treatments and begin to see results, even the most negative people develop amazing levels of positivity and the motivation needed to continue.

A Positive Mental Attitude—More Powerful Than You Can Imagine

Focusing on the physical aspects of scoliosis is the primary method of dealing with the condition, and it's possible these days to do some amazing things to help patients physically. But I'm always amazed by how much a positive mental attitude buoys and strengthens an individual's ability to cope. Patients and loved ones who stay positive and optimistic experience the many joys that life has to offer without letting the reality of scoliosis let them down. They approach treatment with a demeanor that gives them a boost of confidence, which leads to a greater chance of improvement. And they inspire others who may be facing a life with scoliosis.

Yes, we're capable of helping patients reduce their abnormal spinal curvatures here at the Scoliosis Reduction Center. But without the positivity of our patients, our efforts would not be nearly as successful. A positive mental attitude is truly one of the best tools for helping patients find hope and healing. Thankfully, our methods of treatment help patients achieve the results that can fuel positivity.

Five Facts about Pediatric Scoliosis

Scoliosis affects people of all ages, but when the condition is discussed, talk tends to center on adolescents and sometimes adults. However, scoliosis also affects young children, well before they have reached adolescence. This type of scoliosis is known as *pediatric scoliosis.*

Technically, adolescents are in the pediatric phase of their lives, but the way scoliosis affects their bodies is different than how it affects those who have not yet reached adolescence. Additionally, there are numerous lifestyle differences between young children and those who have reached the stage of adolescence. This distinction is important for parents to understand as they move forward and seek treatment options.

What I want to shed light on is what's known as *juvenile early-onset scoliosis,* which occurs in children between the ages of three and ten. It differs from both infantile scoliosis and adolescent scoliosis, even though all fall under the umbrella of pediatric scoliosis. In the case of infantile scoliosis, some data shows that small curves *can* resolve themselves, though no one can be sure which curves will progress and which ones will resolve; consistent management is still recommended. Juvenile early-onset scoliosis is much more likely to progress throughout childhood and well into adulthood with no intervention. That being said, the individuals who have the most growing to do are usually the ones who experience the greatest risk of progression. Scoliosis tends to become worse during periods of physical growth, so it affects younger people who have not yet hit their adolescent growth spurt potentially more than anyone else. That is why pediatric scoliosis—and juvenile early-onset scoliosis, in particular—should be taken very seriously.

Demystifying Scoliosis Progression

Before I get into my five facts about pediatric scoliosis, I think it's important to spend a bit more time demystifying scoliosis progression.

For young people and their parents, scoliosis progression is a fairly mysterious issue. but there are some key factors that can help patients and parents understand it better:

- **Age**—When a child is diagnosed at a younger age, it generally means there's a higher risk of scoliosis curve progression. As I mentioned above, the younger you are, the more you have to grow, which means that the curvature will likely progress more during growth. For children ten years of age or younger, a small curve (between five and nineteen degrees) has a 45 percent chance of progressing. But a curve measuring between twenty and twenty-nine degrees has an almost 100 percent chance of progressing. As children get older, those percentages of likely progression decrease.

- **Skeletal Maturity**—There's a growth indicator known as the *Risser sign* that's visible on X-rays and refers to the level of pelvic calcification as a measure of skeletal maturity. This can be used to demonstrate how much more a child has to grow. It's measured on a scale of zero to five, with a score of five indicating adult maturity levels. The higher the Risser score, generally, the less likely it is that a curve will progress.

- **Gender**—Girls are more likely to experience scoliosis that will progress to the point at which treatment is required. For curvatures that measure greater than 30 degrees, girls are ten times more likely to experience scoliosis progression.

- **Curvature Pattern**—Some curve patterns are more likely to progress than others. For example, a thoracic curve, which is one of the more common patterns to appear, is also one of the more likely to progress.

As you can see, scoliosis progression isn't nearly as mysterious as it might seem initially. While it may be difficult for the average person to understand, doctors and chiropractors who have received scoliosis-specific training are well versed in the nature of progression.

To help you further understand the impact and reality of pediatric scoliosis, here are five facts that should enhance your comprehension of the condition.

Fact #1—Early Diagnosis Is Essential for the Best Outcomes

While this is true for scoliosis patients of any age, it's especially critical for those under the age of ten. Parents need to pay close attention to their children during these crucial years of life and watch for signs of scoliosis such as uneven shoulders or hips. The signs can be subtle, so parents and regular caregivers are uniquely suited to be aware of body changes that could indicate the presence of scoliosis.

When scoliosis is detected early, it can give parents and medical professionals the opportunity to develop the most effective treatment plans. Because abnormal spinal curvatures tend to progress over time, the sooner the condition is detected, the better. And when scoliosis is diagnosed before the crucial age of the first major growth spurt, the potential for healing and reducing curvatures has very few limits.

Keep in mind, though, that early detection does not always guarantee better outcomes. Even when guidelines are followed and observation is done regularly, a lot of progression can happen over the course of a year.

Scoliosis in children is also a pain-free condition, in most cases. Children are unlikely to complain about the effects of an abnormal curvature if they don't feel pain. Nor are they likely to notice changes in their bodies that may indicate the development of the condition. That places the burden on parents to be extra aware of what their children are going through.

Another factor to consider is the reality that children become more private and less likely to reveal aspects of themselves to adults as they get older and approach adolescence. Opportunities to notice the presence of scoliosis dwindle over time as parents stop dressing and bathing their children. A routine exam or checkup may lead to the diagnosis of the condition, but if a parent or caregiver can notice the early signs as soon as possible, diagnosis—and treatment—can happen sooner than later.

Fact #2—Surgery Is Not an Option

In my opinion, surgery for scoliosis should be avoided, if at all possible, in any case. But when it comes to juvenile scoliosis, even the medical establishment agrees with me. Surgery is usually not recommended until a patient reaches the early teen years, after they have experienced their growth spurt. It's best not to perform surgery until the teenage years because surgery at younger ages can be more complicated. It can stunt growth and create conditions where multiple surgeries become necessary.

Fact #3—Observation and Examination Are Standard Treatments

Although the medical establishment will generally not recommend surgery for juvenile scoliosis patients, the traditional treatment path still leads to the operating table. Once the condition has been diagnosed in a child, doctors will usually proceed cautiously, tentatively, and in a manner characterized by inaction instead of action. This entails a great deal of simply watching and waiting, with examinations happening at regularly scheduled intervals. Traditional bracing apparatus are sometimes prescribed in the hopes of stopping a progression, but beyond that, the traditional model of treatment has patients biding their time until their curvatures progress to the point where surgery becomes a justifiable option.

Fact #4—Children with Scoliosis Benefit from an Active Lifestyle

Sports, physical play, and exercise are extraordinarily important for the lives of children with scoliosis. Juvenile patients who avoid physical activity run the risk of losing mobility and strength over time, which decreases the chances of treating the condition effectively. Exercise can increase bone density and make the body healthier overall. This helps with other conditions of the skeletal system, such as osteoporosis, as well. Girls are at a much higher risk of developing osteoporosis than boys, so parents need to be especially encouraging when it comes to sports and exercise for their female children.

Fact #5—Chiropractic-Centered Scoliosis Treatment Can Be Effective for Juvenile Patients

Although no scientific studies have been performed specifically on juvenile patients who experience chiropractic-centered treatment, I can tell you that it's highly effective, based on my experience.

The approach I believe in helps patients avoid surgery later in life, and it ensures that they develop in as healthy a manner as possible. With children, treatment can be quite challenging. They have a long road ahead of them, and the process requires a strong commitment from not only the patients themselves, but also their parents, loved ones, and caregivers. Moreover, children aren't always equipped to understand the nature of scoliosis and the reasons for the treatments they receive.

Nevertheless, the benefits of treating juvenile early-onset scoliosis using the chiropractic-centered approach are potentially tremendous. I urge parents to help their children develop willpower and routines that keep them practicing healthy habits. Yes, watching and waiting may be much easier, and it's endorsed by the traditional model of treatment. But it increases the risk of progression and the likelihood of a surgical recommendation. With the chiropractic-centered approach, we help children and parents avoid expensive and invasive surgical procedures. It's hard work. My patients and I agree that it's well worth the effort, though!

Four Tips for Handling Scoliosis Later in Life

When I talk and write about scoliosis, much of my focus is on adolescents who have the condition. Adolescent idiopathic scoliosis (AIS) is the most commonly known type of the condition, and it becomes evident at a crucial time in a child's life. When the condition is approached proactively and quickly, adolescents have a much better chance of reducing their curvatures and preventing the hardships that can come with dealing with a more pronounced, severe curvature. I'm also focused on helping patients avoid surgery, which is easier to do when I can work with them as soon as possible following a diagnosis.

Scoliosis does not just affect teenagers, though. In some cases, individuals don't discover or develop their scoliosis until after puberty. This is what's known as *adult scoliosis*.

Adult scoliosis can emerge during adulthood, but it's likely that adults with the condition actually had it during adolescence, but it remained undiagnosed and untreated until adulthood.

Regardless of the nature of the condition or how it arose, auu... with scoliosis—especially older adults—must treat the condition differently than younger people with scoliosis.

The Causes of Adult Scoliosis

Occasionally, adult scoliosis is caused by changes in the spine that are experienced after the body has stopped developing. It's thought that the aging process or other degenerative processes might contribute to the development of scoliosis for older individuals.

In other cases, adult scoliosis can be caused by what's known as a *paralytic curve*. This means that the muscles surrounding the spine don't work properly, which can throw the spine out of balance and alignment. Over time, this can lead to the abnormal, paralytic curvature. Often, paralytic curvatures result from spinal cord injuries that precede paralysis. This is extremely rare, though. Similarly, neuromuscular diseases such as cerebral palsy, polio, or muscular dystrophy can also lead to abnormal curvatures in what's known as a *myopathic deformity*. Myopathic, in this case, refers to muscles that don't work properly.

Scoliosis in adults can also be caused by a secondary condition. Osteoporosis, for example, results in the loss of bone mass, which can lead to the compression fractures of the spine, sometimes resulting in scoliosis. It's also possible for surgery to cause an imbalance in the spine that can lead to scoliosis.

These causes are relatively rare in comparison to idiopathic curves, however. Idiopathic adult scoliosis, which is a continuation of adolescent idiopathic scoliosis now progressing in maturity, is by far the most common type. By its nature, there's no easily determined reason or single cause for it. It could be the result of a number of factors. The fact is that it's impossible to tell how most cases of adult scoliosis were caused.

It used to be taught that patients should stop worrying about scoliosis progression once they stopped growing. That turned out to be bad advice. Idiopathic scoliosis can still progress during adulthood. Rates of progression vary, but can be measured anywhere from a half degree to two degrees per year. After about the age of fifty, the rate of progression can increase much more.

The Symptoms of Adult Scoliosis

Adults who discover that they have scoliosis are usually led to the doctor for a diagnosis because they begin to experience one or more common symptoms.

A pronounced lean to one side, uneven shoulder height or the presence of a rib hump are some of the frequently noticed symptoms in adults. Adults may notice several of these symptoms, and they might notice that these symptoms become more pronounced when bending over, which can be an alarming sight.

In adults with scoliosis, back pain can develop and become quite intense. This is one of the major differences between the adolescent version of the condition and the version experienced by older individuals. Teens who develop scoliosis have bodies that are still in stages of growth. Therefore, upward movement is always happening in the spine, which relieves the pressure that would otherwise exist and cause pain. Adults have stopped growing, and their spines have settled due to gravity, which compresses the elements of the spine, often leading to pain. This causes greater pressure on nerves and potentially the entire spinal cord as a scoliosis curve develops and becomes increasingly severe.

In the most severe cases of adult scoliosis, pressure on the spinal cord can lead to deficiencies in coordination and the impairment of the ability to use the limbs. This can make it difficult for patients to walk normally or participate in normal physical activity. Thankfully, these symptoms are rare, but they should be noted as typical differences between adult scoliosis and adolescent scoliosis.

How to Live with Adult Scoliosis— Four Tips for a Better Life

#1—Be Proactive, Not Reactive

Adults with scoliosis don't have the luxury of time that adolescents experience. Their bodies have grown fully, and they're at risk for a continuous progression of their abnormal spinal curvatures. Scoliosis never improves on its own through inaction. Effective treatment must involve active participation by the patient. Obtaining a diagnosis is critical. Then, patients should consult with experts to determine the appropriate next steps.

#2—Get Healthy

Life with scoliosis is easier—and the treatment of scoliosis is easier—when the body and mind are healthy. A scoliosis diagnosis shouldn't prevent an adult of any age from undertaking a fitness regimen. Losing weight, increasing strength, enhancing flexibility, and ceasing bad habits such as smoking can create positive changes in the body that reduce the harmful impacts of scoliosis. A healthy, positive mind-set, as I wrote about in the previous section, is also key to moving forward successfully. Patients respond more favorably to chiropractic-centered treatments, as well, when they make an effort to improve overall health. Of course, it's important to ensure that any exercise regimen is undertaken with the support and guidance of a medical professional. Adults with scoliosis can cause setbacks for themselves if they don't approach getting healthy the right way.

#3—Don't Make Assumptions

Many adults with scoliosis automatically assume that the path that leads to surgery is the only one they can safely walk. Or they may assume that their condition will limit them significantly through the rest of their lives. These assumptions aren't necessarily true. While the medical establishment leads patients down the path toward surgery more often than not, it's not inevitable. In fact, I would encourage those with adult scoliosis to be very skeptical of the benefits of surgery while exploring alternative options for treatment.

#4—Consider the Chiropractic-Centered
Approach to Scoliosis Treatment

As a leading scoliosis chiropractor, I work with patients of all ages with varying degrees of severity. I see younger people improve and actually reduce their curvatures on a regular basis. It may surprise you, but I also see similar progress in my adult patients. The chiropractic-centered approach to scoliosis treatment is proactive and designed to help patients avoid invasive, expensive surgery. It requires a commitment from the patient to work hard and participate enthusiastically in the various aspects of the approach. But it works—and it changes lives for the better, even for those who previously thought that their adult scoliosis was untreatable without surgery.

Hope for Adult Scoliosis

We live in a culture that looks to youth for a promise of what's possible in the future. When it comes to treating scoliosis, the focus on youth remains in the writing, literature, and discussion of the condition. But that doesn't mean adults can't experience relief. Older individuals with scoliosis should live with just as much hope as their younger counterparts. It's my job to keep giving them reasons to do so. And I think the positive results I've experienced with my patients speak for themselves.

Life with Scoliosis Is Different Than You Might Think!

The advice, wisdom, and guidance I've given here in this chapter should shed a light on scoliosis from a perspective of hope. Sadly, the talk surrounding scoliosis does not feature much hopefulness or positivity. Patients, parents, family members, and loved ones shouldn't have to endure life dealing with the condition thinking that expensive, invasive surgery is the only option for attempting to reduce or relieve scoliosis. People can live amazing, productive, and active lives with scoliosis. I know because I see them every day in my practice. They're my patients, my partners, and my colleagues, and I couldn't do what I do without them.

Ultimately, you shouldn't automatically buy the conventional wisdom about scoliosis just because it seems authoritative. Much of society's attitude toward the condition was developed decades ago and has rarely been questioned since. I know that there are new ways to face the condition and approach its treatment.

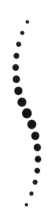

CHAPTER FOUR

Diet, Exercise, Lifestyle, and Scoliosis

IN THE PREVIOUS CHAPTER, I explored aspects of life with scoliosis and provided some wisdom and guidance designed to improve people's experience with the condition. There are many ways in which a person can live life with scoliosis, and with the right guidance, a person's life can be incredibly rich and fulfilling. It's also crucial to understand that modern, alternative approaches to treatment are more than just promising—they're demonstrably effective.

As I mention frequently throughout this book, treatment of scoliosis tends to be easier and more effective when it's approached proactively and in a healthy manner. Patients who come to me and my staff with an already healthy lifestyle that features a good diet and proper exercise tend to perform much better in treatment. They're more optimistic and less prone to emotional turbulence. They respond to treatment with a winning attitude. Furthermore, they're much better prepared for the physical and mental demands of the treatment process.

As you read this chapter, I invite you to consider how diet, exercise, and lifestyle choices impact your life, whether you have scoliosis or you care for someone with the condition. How have your choices benefited you? How have they impacted you negatively? What were your choices like during the time in your life when you were happiest and most fulfilled?

Diet, exercise, and lifestyle are critical factors to consider for everyone. And as you reflect on your own life, I'm sure you'll come to realize just how much choices in these areas create ripple effects throughout the years and throughout the many aspects of your existence. For scoliosis patients, these impacts are amplified, which is why this chapter is so important.

Yoga for Scoliosis—Can It Really Make a Difference?

Yoga is an ancient practice with roots that go back more than five thousand years to India. But its popularity has exploded in the last decade or two, especially in Western countries like the United States. People who practice yoga experience a number of benefits, many of which are now backed by science (Healthline, 2017). It can relieve stress and anxiety, reduce inflammation, improve flexibility and balance, increase strength, and much more.

What about yoga for scoliosis, though? Is it an effective treatment?

The traditional orthopedic method of treatment—consisting of observation, bracing, and surgery—is well established, but it's far from the only approach available. These days, patients and parents are becoming increasingly aware of alternative treatments, many of which are capable of creating significant improvements. Yoga for scoliosis is just one alternative element of treatment that people consider, and it seems promising considering the benefits it provides to those who practice. But is it truly helpful for people who have abnormally curved spines?

The Potential Benefits of Yoga for Scoliosis

Yoga is a terrific form of exercise for certain types of muscles, particularly type-one, slow-twitch muscles. Most yoga poses involve long, isometric contractions that involve holding a specific position or pose for a long period of time. For most people, this is highly beneficial to spinal strength. Furthermore, the muscles that are typically strengthened by yoga are those that affect posture. So, in this sense, yoga can be effective.

I honestly believe that yoga can help people with pain, posture, and the ways in which they carry themselves. It's an absolutely effective mode of exercise in that regard. But it's important for people to understand that yoga, in and of itself, isn't an effective sole treatment for the reduction of scoliosis.

Certainly, if a patient works with a yoga instructor who understands scoliosis—and understands each specific case of the condition—it *can* be an effective form of exercise to maintain fitness. Unfortunately, most yoga instructors and practitioners don't make special considerations for people who have abnormal spinal curvatures.

An Issue of Symmetry

In most cases, yoga is practiced in a symmetrical manner. Basically, it's performed in a way that assumes one side of the body is a perfect mirror image of the other. But we know that for people with scoliosis, this isn't the case. Therefore, when it comes to reducing curvatures, yoga is simply not effective. It does not do anything specific to help reduce a scoliosis curve.

By the time a person is able to perform yoga well, severe asymmetrical motion has occurred in the spine. Essentially, the spine isn't moving the same in both directions, which can exacerbate the issues associated with the condition. Imagine that you want to work and strengthen both of your bicep muscles in your upper arms. However, one elbow is only capable of a very limited range of motion, while the other is capable of normal motion. In this scenario, only the bicep on the arm with a normal range of motion will get an effective workout, even with the identical set of exercises. Yoga for scoliosis has a similar effect on the muscles surrounding the spine: on one side, a patient may be capable of normal motion, but on the other, they may be severely restricted, which will have negative impact.

Once a person has received a scoliosis diagnosis, yoga is minimally effective in reducing a curve size, and this is because of the asymmetrical joint motion. At this point, the condition has become structural, and there's very little—if anything—that the practice of yoga can do to restore motion or reduce curvatures.

Additionally, depending upon curve type and severity, yoga can actually make some of the common symptoms worse.

I don't mean to give yoga a bad name! I honestly believe that it can be incredibly helpful for building strength, flexibility and range of motion. It's just not effective as a treatment to reduce scoliosis.

Scoliosis-Specific Exercises

Scoliosis-specific exercise, on the other hand, is a form of alternative treatment that can help patients experience a number of benefits—particularly when combined with scoliosis-specific chiropractic, therapy, and specialized bracing.

Scoliosis-specific exercises are customized for each individual curve type as well as each patient's ability to perform the exercises.

A ten-year-old with a fifty-degree curve would be given a completely different set of exercises than a twenty-year-old with an identical curve, for example. Someone who is fifty years old with the identical curve would also require their own customized set of exercises.

For example, I could have a five-year-old patient with a curve that's technically appropriate for a variety of exercises. But I have to take into account that she's only five years old, which means that I have to prescribe exercises that can be easily guided by her parents in order to have the desired effect. However, if I had a twelve-year-old patient with the same curve, the exercises may be different.

Age is just one factor of many that should be considered when devising a scoliosis-specific exercise regimen.

The only way to know for sure if an exercise or fitness program is appropriate is to have the spine assessed by an expert who can take curve type, curve size, abilities, and a host of other factors into account.

The Truth about Yoga for Scoliosis

Yoga is one of the most beneficial forms of exercise available, and its five-thousand-year track record speaks for itself. It provides a wide range of science-backed benefits to those who practice, and it can be incredibly useful in the quest for greater physical and mental fitness. That being said, it's not an effective alternative treatment for reducing scoliosis. Yes, it can be great for physical fitness, but getting in shape and reducing a curve are two different things.

In most cases, scoliosis patients can experience benefits from exercise, stretching, and other types of physical activity. Depending on the person and their specific curve, there may even be some yoga poses that relieve pain and improve flexibility. But I can't recommend yoga as a treatment, especially if it's not practiced under the guidance of someone who fully understands the condition.

Scoliosis and Diet: Four Foods to Add to Your Grocery List

To the average person, a special scoliosis diet may not seem necessary. But for those who are faced with a scoliosis diagnosis, diet becomes an important factor for recovery, building strength, living with more energy, and improving overall health and wellness. A properly calibrated diet will not heal scoliosis or reduce curvature by itself; however, it will help create conditions within the body that are much more conducive to healing and the reduction of the negative aspects of scoliosis. And when the appropriate scoliosis diet is introduced along with a treatment plan that focuses on strengthening the spine and improving function, it can have a tremendous positive impact.

Why Do Diet and Nutrition Matter for Scoliosis?

When I see scoliosis patients and develop plans for their treatment, I always address the condition from a structural standpoint first. Correcting the abnormal curvature of the spine is always my top priority, so we always get to work on the structural aspect of the condition right away. That being said, diet and nutrition enter the picture soon after we begin to address structural issues.

Nutrition is very important for scoliosis patients for a variety of reasons:

- leaner patients respond more positively to treatments (chiropractic, therapy, exercise, and corrective bracing), particularly those who are adolescent patients.
- There are links between a deficiency of neurotransmitters and the development of scoliosis; by introducing precursors to neurotransmitters (such as amino acids) into the

diet, the body can produce them naturally, which may have a significantly positive impact on the condition.

- Many scoliosis patients are unable to methylate the vitamin B12 effectively. Methylation is an essential biological process that helps the body produce neurotransmitters such as serotonin and dopamine. To improve this process, patients can take methylated B12, which can boost production of neurotransmitters. It's worth introducing into a diet because of the potential improvements it can provide; if it does *not* stimulate the production of neurotransmitters, no harm is done.

- The proper diet leads to greater overall health. When a patient feels better as a result of a healthier diet, they tend to take other aspects of their health more seriously, which leads to improvements in all areas of well-being. Patients begin to see results they like, and they become more committed to a healthy diet and more likely to buy into the overall course of treatment.

- Scoliosis is associated with lower bone density; by introducing a combination of special minerals and trace elements into the diet, overall bone health and strength can be improved.

- A healthy diet helps patients reduce the likelihood they will suffer from chronic inflammation, which can lead to a loss of bone density, which can increase the likelihood of pain.

Foods Scoliosis Patients Must Avoid

Convenience and cost have become the primary drivers of diet, particularly here in the United States. Bad nutrition has become part of the culture, and it has produced an unhealthy populace, in general.

Food items that are loaded with sugar, salt, and unhealthy fats are cheap and easy to find. But they're the enemy of a proper scoliosis diet!

Some examples of foods scoliosis patients should avoid include the following:

- fast food or other highly processed varieties of junk food
- soda pop (even the diet varieties)
- foods containing corn syrup in any form (high fructose, crystallized, etc.)
- artificial sweeteners like Equal, Splenda, Saccharin, Nutrasweet, and others
- soy milk and other soy products
- pasteurized milk
- MSG (also known as Monosodium Glutamate)
- excessive salt (sea salt is preferred)
- sugar (Stevia is a good substitute)
- alcohol
- coffee
- white flour
- chocolate (though dark chocolate is okay in limited quantities)

For many people, the items and ingredients listed above will be difficult to remove from the diet, which is understandable given their availability and popularity. But switching to a healthier diet is well worth the effort.

I suggest making dietary switches slowly at first. Psychologically speaking, it's easier for people to deal with gradual changes than an abrupt and complete overhaul of the diet. It also increases the likelihood that dietary changes will become permanent.

Four Foods to Focus on for the Proper Scoliosis Diet

Now that I've listed foods that should *not* be consumed by those with scoliosis, let's get to the good stuff!

The following food items provide excellent nutrition and improve the body's ability to recover successfully from scoliosis. They promote greater strength, stamina, and energy, which helps scoliosis patients build more active and capable bodies. And they're excellent for everyone, regardless of whether they deal with scoliosis or not—the whole family can get on board!

#1—Fresh Fruits and Vegetables

Fresh fruits and vegetables are packed with nutrients that are crucial for the health and maintenance of the human body. They also contain fiber, which is something that's sorely lacking from most diets. Additionally, the consumption of fresh fruits and vegetables can contribute to a reduced risk of chronic diseases.

The list of healthy fruits and vegetables is a long one, but here are some items you can add to your cart the next time you go grocery shopping:

- broccoli
- apples
- tomatoes
- avocado
- cauliflower
- carrots
- kale
- brussels sprouts
- oranges
- pears
- peaches

- celery
- green beans

Remember—these items should be purchased fresh, not frozen. However, frozen vegetables are better for the body than anything on the list of foods to avoid. Also, juicing fruits isn't as healthy as you might think. Juicing removes fiber and concentrates sugars. And if you buy premade juices, chances are they're loaded with added sugar, too.

Not sure what to do with all these fruits and veggies? The internet is full of healthy recipes that bring out the best of these items. Fruits and veggies also make great snacks, especially when paired with healthy hummus or nut butters!

#2—Unprocessed Meats

Chicken, turkey, beef, fish, and other meats provide essential protein to the body. Just be sure to avoid oily or fried meats, like those you would get at a fast-food restaurant. You should also steer clear of packaged lunch meats and pork, which contain preservatives and other unhealthy add-ons.

#3—Foods Containing Calcium and Vitamin D

Calcium, which is utilized in conjunction with magnesium and many other trace minerals, is a highly important mineral in the human body. It's crucial for scoliosis patients to introduce into their diets via supplements or whole foods. Poppy, sesame, celery, and chia seeds all contain high amounts of calcium (in addition to super-healthy proteins and fats). Beans and lentils also contain calcium, as well as a number of other important minerals. If you're looking for a healthy snack, almonds are excellent, too.

Vitamin D is also crucial, largely because many people don't get enough of it. Supplements are helpful, but vitamin D can also be found in several foods, including fish, eggs, and mushrooms. Sunlight also stimulates the body's production of vitamin D. In today's world, most people don't get enough of it, though, which is one of the reasons people's vitamin D levels tend to be so low.

#4—Water

While it's not technically a food, water is critical in the ideal scoliosis diet. Proper hydration keeps all the body's systems in top working order, and it aids in most of the body's natural processes.

Water is also the perfect substitute for soda, coffee, alcoholic beverages, and other unhealthy drinks. I suggest increasing your consumption of water by keeping a bottle or glass of it near you at all times. It quenches thirst better than soda, and it can even stave off hunger pangs that might otherwise lead you to eating unhealthy snacks!

A Challenge Worth Taking On

I get that changing your family's diet may seem impossible if you're accustomed to eating certain foods regularly. But the benefits of altering your nutrition are profound. You don't have to change the way you eat overnight; simply start by making small changes. You or your child will feel better and more motivated to make further changes, which will boost energy and strength. Doing so will also significantly impact your ability—or your child's ability—to treat scoliosis effectively.

Four Scoliosis Exercises That Really Work

If you ask the average person about scoliosis exercises, they might respond with a confused look. To most people, scoliosis is seen as a limiting condition that prevents patients from participating in physical activities. They may see scoliosis patients as fragile individuals who must be kept away from activities like exercise or sports.

For those who live with scoliosis, however, exercise is a crucial component of treating the condition.

Participating in sports and other forms of exercise helps patients—especially adolescents—develop well-being in a variety of aspects of life. It helps them realize that life does not have to be limited by their diagnosis. All you have to do is take a look at the accomplishments of Usain Bolt to realize that physical activity can have a remarkably positive impact.

Furthermore, exercise and participation in sports aids in treatment by increasing strength, flexibility, and overall health. Many parents come to me assuming that I will recommend for their child to stop playing sports and are surprised when I encourage them to continue their participation. Staying active and engaging in exercise makes the whole body healthier, which in turn leads to more positive outcomes for scoliosis treatment.

Sports and Scoliosis

I want to get into some specific scoliosis exercises that can benefit patients, but first I'd like to address participation in sports, especially for adolescents with scoliosis.

Personally, participation in sports has been one of the most gratifying aspects of my life. Once I got well during my youth, sports taught me a lot about my own body, and they helped guide me down the path that led me to where I am today. Sports provide a great way for adolescents to express themselves, build relationships, achieve goals, and learn the value of a commitment to fitness.

But not all sports are appropriate for those with scoliosis. Specifically, any sport or activity that promotes thoracic extension (a flattening in the mid-back area) should be avoided.

Swimming is often recommended as the best sport to participate in for those with scoliosis. The water simulates a weightless environment, which places less impact on the spine and can improve the health of the spinal discs. It also utilizes a wide range of the body's muscles, providing a highly balanced form of activity. It's not without its potential dangers, though. Some swimming techniques can promote hyperextension (a flattening of the middle back), so it's important to remain mindful.

Running and walking are also great for scoliosis patients, as is hiking. Sprinting (Usain Bolt's specialty) is probably better for the spine than long-distance running. Cross-country skiing is also a wonderful physical activity for adolescents with scoliosis.

Collision sports don't need to be prohibited entirely, but they should be approached with caution. Football, hockey, soccer, gymnastics and other similar sports are more likely to cause injury to the spine or possibly reduce the effectiveness of a treatment plan. Adolescents with scoliosis should probably avoid these types of sports if they want the best possible outcomes from treatment. They should also steer clear of sports that involve the use of one side of the body more than the other (such as golf, bowling, or tennis).

Repetitive shocks are characteristic of some sports like weight lifting, long-distance running, the long jump, or horseback riding. Therefore, they may increase compressive forces applied to the spine, and should be approached with caution.

The great news about the chiropractic-centered approach is that when a patient complies with corrective treatment, they condition the body in such a way as to lift many of the restrictions that would otherwise impede them. Under the chiropractic-centered model, restrictions are rarely placed on patients for the long term.

Scoliosis-Specific Exercises

Patients who come here to the Scoliosis Reduction Center receive treatment in a few key categories, one of which is scoliosis-specific exercise. Scoliosis-specific exercises—SSEs—are customized for each patient based on the individual's ability and curve type. They involve reflexive exercises, movement-based exercise, and isometric exercises.

With a skilled instructor guiding them, patients can incorporate SSEs into activities they already enjoy. This allows them to help ensure they help the scoliosis instead of possibly making it worse.

Each patient is evaluated and given a set of exercises designed specifically for them. Additionally, they're given a specific program involving therapy, chiropractic care, and corrective bracing, as prescribed. When all aspects are combined, it creates a powerful approach to treatment that delivers real, measurable improvements.

Four Scoliosis Exercises That Can Benefit Patients

Now I want to tell you about a few scoliosis exercises that can be performed by most patients to good effect.

First, it's important to know that you shouldn't begin any sort of exercise or physical fitness program without consulting your doctor or trusted medical professional. Because every patient is different, it's critical each individual approach exercise in a manner consistent with their unique abilities and spinal curvature.

That being said, here are some of the best exercises for those with scoliosis.

#1—Stretching

Stretches that can be done in a symmetrical manner can relieve tension and tightness in the muscles. Some examples include the child's pose, chest and shoulder stretches, and hip flexion stretches.

#2—Rowing

Rowing works and strengthens the *latissimus dorsi* back muscles, and there are many ways to do it. You can sit on a stability ball while facing a pulley machine, or use rowing-specific equipment.

#3—The Plank

Planking is a deceptively simple way to strengthen the body's core and improve strength. You can begin by placing your forearms and knees on the ground, with your elbows beneath your shoulders. Hold the position for as long as you feel comfortable. If you feel ready for a bigger challenge, lift your knees off the floor and stabilize yourself with your toes. When you plank properly, you will feel it in your lower abdominal muscles and your lower back. If you feel any pinching or pain, adjust your body or stop performing the exercise until you can receive the proper guidance.

#4—CLEAR Institute Back Exercises

As a CLEAR (Chiropractic, Leadership, Educational, Advancement, and Research) certified doctor, I stand behind the recommendations of the organization and their comprehensive list of back exercises. These exercises can be performed in almost any setting, and they can provide increased strength and relief when done properly.

A Note about Exercising Carefully

Exercise can provide serious, highly impactful benefits for those with scoliosis, but patients and parents need to approach exercise thoughtfully. No exercise program should be approached without first consulting a doctor, and any exercise that causes pain or discomfort should be ceased and reevaluated before continuing.

Scoliosis Massage: Is It an Effective Treatment?

When the average person feels strain, discomfort, aches, or pains, it's not unusual for them to seek relief in the form of massage. Skilled massage practitioners understand the human body in unique and valuable ways. This gives them the ability to locate the source of tension and ease it through their specialized techniques. And for many people, massage is the ideal treatment for those times when they feel tight, stressed, and tense.

But what about scoliosis massage? Since massage can be so effective at providing relief for bodily tension and stress, it would seem that it might also provide relief for those who have scoliosis. This makes sense. The discomfort experienced by individuals with scoliosis often arrives in the form of tension in the muscles, therefore, it stands to reason that massage would be an effective treatment. However, the efficacy of scoliosis massage isn't so simply understood.

Yes, scoliosis massage can be effective, but it's important for patients and loved ones to understand how massage should complement a comprehensive treatment program before they proceed.

Are you a scoliosis patient or the parent of a child with scoliosis? I can understand why you may be considering scoliosis massage. It's normal for you to be exploring all the numerous treatments and procedures that are available. I applaud your desire to be proactive with the condition, but I also want to ensure that you make the best, most well-informed decisions. Scoliosis massage can provide relief and help the healing process, but it's critical that you approach it with the right knowledge and mind-set.

Following are some of the things you should keep in mind as you consider scoliosis massage.

Scoliosis Is Strictly Structural—Not Muscular

By the time scoliosis is diagnosed, the muscles are reacting to the structural component, which impacts the muscles, not the other way around.

Fundamentally, massage can't actually heal or correct scoliosis. Yes, it can provide relief, but in and of itself, it's not an approach that improves or reduces the curve. The reason is that scoliosis is a condition of the structure of the spine, while massage is a technique that works the body's muscles.

An individual who has scoliosis can benefit from massage because their muscles may be overly tense and tight from compensating for the abnormal spinal curvature. Muscles perform extra work when they act against the continued progression of the scoliosis. This can lead to a significant amount of discomfort, which can be eased through massage.

It's important to note that tightness and soreness aren't necessarily negative aspects. In many cases, the tightness and soreness come from the muscles acting completely appropriately, given the presence of scoliosis. So I would say that doing scoliosis massage might be useful, but it shouldn't necessarily be done to reduce tightness in the muscles.

Here at the Scoliosis Reduction Center, we utilize percussion therapies, which can simulate massage, in our treatment approach. But this type of therapy isn't a centerpiece. Rather, it's something we use to help patients ease the soreness and fatigue they may feel from therapy or rehab.

Symmetry and Order

Before engaging in scoliosis massage, it's also important to understand when and how it's most effective.

Most of the time, massage is performed symmetrically. This means that the provider will generally work different areas of the body with equal pressure and duration. The left side receives the same treatment as the right, in other words. Why is this important to know? Because scoliosis is, by its nature, an asymmetrical condition. Symmetrical massage is appropriate for people who have normal spinal curvatures, but it can present problems for those with scoliosis.

In order to receive the biggest benefit from scoliosis massage, it needs to be performed in a way that takes into account the asymmetry of the individual's spine. Sadly, most massage practitioners don't consider this.

When scoliosis is present, it's normal for muscles on one side of the spine to contract more while the other side may feel more relaxed. This isn't a cause of scoliosis, but a normal reaction of the body designed to help support a curve and keep it upright against the force of gravity. So using massage in an attempt to make the muscles symmetrical may not be the best approach. The imbalances are the body's way of supporting the asymmetrical spine; they may be contracting to prevent further scoliosis progression. Therefore, trying to achieve muscular symmetry without addressing the structural cause normally will not lead to any correction.

Another aspect to take seriously is the order in which massage is provided to a patient. When treating scoliosis, the sequence of treatments is crucial. If massage is administered at the wrong time, it can set patients back and even cause additional pain, strain, or discomfort. But if it's administered at the proper point within treatment, it can provide tremendous relief and aid in the overall treatment process.

Working Together to Treat Scoliosis Effectively

One of the most appealing aspects of receiving treatment here at the Scoliosis Reduction Center is the fact that we perform a full suite of treatments on site. We can ensure the proper approach and the right sequence to help patients reduce their abnormal spinal curvatures. That being said, I understand if a patient wishes to augment their treatments with those provided by outside specialists such as massage therapists.

If you're interested in scoliosis massage, I would advise you to ask your provider if they're willing to work with a scoliosis specialist. Working together, providers can devise the most appropriate treatment techniques, ensuring that everything that's done is done in the best interest of the patient. A scoliosis chiropractor, for example, can offer guidance, making sure that the massage practitioner understands the comprehensive nature of treatment and the asymmetrical reality of the condition.

Is scoliosis massage an effective treatment? By itself, it's not likely to provide long-term relief or healing. But if it's done in the right sequence and with the proper understanding of scoliosis, it can be a useful technique.

Are Our Devices Making Scoliosis Worse?

Today's technology allows us to do some amazing things. For example, I'm writing this on my computer and you may be reading this on a device or you may have purchased the book online. You may be thousands of miles away, but because of the technology involved, you have an opportunity to read this book from the comfort of wherever you happen to be located. Amazing, isn't it?

Technology also helps me evaluate, diagnose, and treat scoliosis patients. Old-school technologies like X-rays are used in conjunction with the most up-to-date scanning and imaging tools to help determine the nature and progress of each patient's condition. Thanks to technological innovations, I'm able to treat more patients more effectively than would have been possible even just five or ten years ago.

We live in an amazing world of innovation, don't we? But we also recognize that there's a dark side to technology. And it affects the lives of scoliosis patients in ways that shouldn't be ignored.

Understanding Ergonomics

When I evaluate and treat my patients, I don't just look at them physically. Scoliosis is a condition that affects numerous aspects of a patient's life, which means that I have to consider their emotional and practical realities as well.

Ergonomics is a term that rarely gets mentioned in traditional scoliosis treatment circles, but it's very important to the chiropractic-centered model of treatment. In case you aren't familiar, ergonomics is defined as the study of people's efficiency in their working environment. I would expand the definition to include all the ways in which people interact with the physical world on a day-to-day basis. Adolescents with scoliosis, for example, may not be dealing with jobs or conditions that are typical in normal working environments. But they go to school, play sports, and interact with the rest of the world and its elements every day. Therefore, ergonomics is something that everyone touched by scoliosis should consider.

The way people interact with their devices also falls under the category of ergonomics. Perhaps it's no surprise to you, but data seems to indicate that smartphone and tablet usage has contributed to increases in reports of neck and back pain. As it turns out, the ways in which people use their devices have major impacts on physical health.

For people with scoliosis, ergonomic considerations are amplified because of the nature of their abnormally curved spines. They're more likely to experience pain and discomfort than those who don't have scoliosis. There are critical times in the lives of scoliosis patients, especially when they're in adolescence and still in the midst of developing physically. Ergonomics are crucial to consider during these times because it's possible that certain activities can make the condition worse, especially when the patient isn't engaged in treatment aimed at reducing the curve.

To me, it's important to have a strong sense of awareness about ergonomics so patients can recognize behaviors that may impact the condition negatively. For young people with scoliosis in today's world, many of those behaviors revolve around device usage.

Ergonomic Advice for Smarter Device Usage

I previously asked if our devices are making scoliosis worse. I have to be honest—we don't really know if this is the case. We may never be able to answer this question conclusively. The fact is that most cases of scoliosis are idiopathic and are likely caused by a host of different factors. There's simply no way to tell with certainty if device usage has an impact on scoliosis. Nevertheless, I think it's important to be aware of physical behaviors and habits so patients can engage in activities in ways that don't pose threats to their health or well-being.

We also don't know exactly how much working with patients ergonomically can improve the condition. We feel confident that it has a positive influence, but we don't know how strong that influence may be. Regardless, I believe strongly in encouraging behaviors that support healthy spines, decrease pain, and enhance physical ability. When patients are smarter with their spines, the treatments provided under the chiropractic-centered model have a greater likelihood of succeeding.

Since devices like smartphones and tablets are so commonly used, especially among adolescents, a lot of media coverage has centered around conditions like *text neck* or *Blackberry thumbs*. These aren't necessarily medically recognized conditions, but I think we all understand that regular usage of devices can have negative physical impacts. And although the long-term implications of device usage aren't known at this time, it's better to err on the side of spine health and safety, particularly for those with scoliosis.

With that in mind, here are some tips that can help scoliosis patients avoid injury, complications, or pain.

- **Hold devices at chest level, not waist level**—Much of the strain that comes from device usage has to do with where people hold their phones. Instead of constantly looking downward, users should raise their phones higher so they can keep their spines straighter and better aligned.

- **Use hands to hold the phone**—This may seem obvious until you realize how often people hold their phones between their shoulders and ears, in addition to other places! Cradling the phone in this fashion puts unnecessary strain and stress on the spine. These days there's no excuse for holding the phone improperly. Users can talk using speakerphone technology or by utilizing any of the many hands-free devices that are available.

- **Avoid typing long passages on smartphone screens**—While it's possible to write an entire novel on a smartphone, our bodies don't react well to extensive typing on tiny phone screens. While phones are fine for texting and short email communications, longer passages of text should be written with proper keyboards. Users should focus on sitting with the proper posture, screen distance, and foot and hand placement. Feet should be flat on the floor. The back should be supported by a chair. Shoulders should be relaxed. Wrists should be in a neutral position.

- **Practice proper placement while reading on a tablet**—It is becoming increasingly common for people to read books on their tablet devices. Sadly, people rarely consider posture, placement, and positioning while doing so. The tablet should be placed in a manner that allows for comfortable body positioning. For those who like to read in bed, propping the tablet up on a pillow can be helpful.

- **Take frequent, extended breaks from devices**—This is probably the most important advice I can give on this subject. Device usage isn't conducive to healthy behaviors for the spine, even if the user is hypervigilant about proper posture and positioning. Frequent breaks and time spent engaging with the world in other ways helps the body retain its flexibility and reduces strain.

Being Smarter with Smart Devices

If you or your child has scoliosis, you can benefit tremendously by paying attention to ergonomics, especially where devices like smartphones and tablets are concerned. Although we can't prove if devices make scoliosis worse, we know that recovering from scoliosis is easier when the body feels healthy, strong, and free from soreness. Therefore, being smart with smartphones and other devices is something I recommend strongly.

Three Reasons Why Active Teens Make Better Scoliosis Patients

In the previous section, I wrote about the realities of life with our smart devices. Now I think it's important to spend some time on the people we tend to associate with smart-device usage—teens. Specifically, I think it's useful to consider how devices and other distractions keep teens and other young people from active lifestyles.

While smart devices may be relatively new, they're just the latest in a long line of items and inventions that keep people from engaging in physical activity. When television entered the picture in the middle of the twentieth century, parents and others became concerned about how it would impact the lives of younger individuals. They feared that the new invention would contribute to an idle, less-active lifestyle. And you know what? People were not wrong when they expressed their concerns over the impact television would have!

Later, video games became incredibly popular, further alarming adults who had concerns about their children's ability to live active, healthy lives. While game makers often boasted that their products positively benefited hand-eye coordination, it became evident over time that video games were keeping kids glued to the couch more than ever. Sure, they were developing their hand-eye coordination, but while they were doing so, they sacrificed the benefits that they would have experienced by engaging in physical play out in the real world.

Now our world is filled with smart devices like cell phones and tablets. It seems like distractions have taken over as the main event in the lives of young people, and it's more challenging than ever before to encourage teens to live active lives.

It is easy to blame TV, video games, and devices for a lack of interest in physical activity. But those things aren't going away anytime soon—or ever! In today's environment, it's necessary for parents to be firm and establish strong boundaries when it comes to how their children interact with devices and other distractions. Yes, it can be challenging to get teens to put down their phones and other devices. But the rewards are considerable, especially for teens who have scoliosis.

Shouldn't Teens with Scoliosis Be More Cautious with Physical Activity?

Before I get into the three reasons why active teens make better scoliosis patients, I would like to debunk the myth that says teens should be treated as if they're extremely fragile if they have scoliosis.

Yes, teens and their parents should approach sports and other types of physical activity with caution. But worries about the impacts of exercise and other more intense body movements can mostly be placed on the back burner. Scoliosis shouldn't be ignored. But it also shouldn't be used as an excuse for a sedentary lifestyle.

Every case of scoliosis is different, just as every individual is different. Therefore, something that affects one teen positively may have a negative impact on a different person. While exercise and activity should be encouraged, it shouldn't be done until a parent has consulted with a medical professional or chiropractor who understands scoliosis.

We want to make sure that teens are given the best possible set of opportunities to live their lives to the fullest and reach their potential. But we also want to give them the best odds at stabilizing—and reducing—their abnormal spinal curvatures while helping them avoid surgery. It can be a balancing act, but that doesn't mean adolescents should avoid activity. In fact, the reality is quite the opposite of that.

Why Do Active Teens Respond Better to Scoliosis Treatment?

Scoliosis is a condition of the spine, but it affects all areas of the body. It even affects non-physical aspects like mood and emotions. In order to treat the condition effectively, it's important to not only look at the spine, but also to examine how the condition manifests in the muscles, nerves and virtually every other system of the anatomy. Generally speaking, physical activity leads to stronger, more flexible bodies, which in turn leads to conditions that are far more conducive to successful treatment.

To get more specific with how physical activity enables the healing process, here are three reasons why active teens make better scoliosis patients.

#1—Active Teens Have a Flexibility Advantage

Scoliosis is often associated with rigidity and stiffness, but there's no reason why those with scoliosis can't be flexible and limber in their bodies. Greater flexibility allows teen patients to respond more favorably to scoliosis-specific exercises and physical therapy, which can lead to a quicker response to treatment. When adolescents with scoliosis come to me with bodies that are used to physical activity, it's easier to integrate them into the treatment program and begin to do the work that will reduce their curvatures.

#2—Active Teens Are Stronger

The treatments that I find most effective are truly remarkable. I've seen patients make incredible progress when they commit to their treatment through ups, downs, and hardships. It takes a certain amount of strength and stamina, both physically and mentally, to participate in the chiropractic-centered approach to scoliosis treatment. We make sure everyone gets up to speed with their abilities to undergo treatment, but those who come to us with a baseline of physical strength and stamina have a definite head start. Their muscles respond much more favorably, and they're better able to endure the more challenging aspects of therapy. Exercise and sports make younger bodies stronger, and greater strength allows patients to get on a faster track to the eventual reduction of their curvatures.

#3—Active Teens Have a Mental Edge

Sports and other types of physical activity aid the body in becoming stronger and more flexible, but they also have an effect on the mind. Anyone who exercises regularly will tell you that they get a mood boost whenever they work out—the so-called *runner's high* is just one example of this effect. For teens, staying active absolutely impacts mood and mental ability in a positive fashion. Active adolescents tend to be more focused, energetic and happier. They're tuned in to the positive effects of engaging in physical activity, and they're aware of the rewards that come from pushing their bodies through exercise. Furthermore, sports can help teens develop a healthy competitive attitude, which comes in handy during treatment.

Ultimately, active teens benefit considerably from exercise and participation in sports. They respond to treatment much more favorably than their less-active counterparts, and generally approach treatment with a can-do attitude. Being active gives them an edge mentally, physically, and in terms of flexibility, but it also helps them understand their own bodies. Sure, there are risks involved in sports and other physical activities, but that's true for people whether they have scoliosis or not. To me, active teens are ideal patients, so I encourage you to do what you can to get your son or daughter off their device and onto the playing field!

What Is the Right Activity Level for Scoliosis Patients?

Teens with scoliosis experience a number of important benefits from living active lives. Adults with scoliosis can also enhance their lives through physical activity. But because every individual—and every case of scoliosis—is unique, there's no one-size-fits-all exercise regimen that's appropriate for people with the condition.

Determining the appropriate activity level for someone with scoliosis is critical to their ability to treat the condition successfully. Too much inactivity leads to a decrease in flexibility and muscular strength. This makes it much more difficult to treat scoliosis. On the other hand, too much physical activity (or the wrong *type* of physical activity) can be equally harmful to those with scoliosis.

So, how can individuals with scoliosis establish an exercise/activity level that maximizes the benefits of physical activity while preventing harm to the body? It all depends.

Adolescent Patients versus Mature Patients

There are major differences between the experience of having scoliosis as a teen and the reality of having the condition as an adult.

The most obvious difference is that teens with scoliosis have bodies that are still growing and developing. Physically, they may be awkward and unsure of themselves, but they have the energy and vitality of youth on their side. Their bodies respond very well to physical activity, and they tend to recover more quickly after periods of exertion. They're also much less limited by pain, thanks to the upward, uncompressed direction of growth in their spines.

Adults with scoliosis have bodies that have seen more wear and tear. They have stopped growing and have generally settled into the shape that they will take for the rest of their lives. While most of the body remains static—apart from the changes brought on by the natural aging process—the spine will continue to progress its abnormal curvature. Curvatures that have existed since childhood can become severe in adulthood without intervention, and the progression of the curvature can negatively impact the person's ability to participate in physical activity.

Striking the Right Balance

In both cases, it's necessary to find the appropriate level of activity. Active bodies respond better to treatment, whereas sedentary bodies are weaker, less responsive to treatment, and more prone to injury. Eliminating physical activity shouldn't be a real consideration unless the individual is in an extreme state of pain and/or fragility.

The goal is to find the correct level of activity for each patient. The goal is to reduce risk of injury or setback while doing enough to add strength and agility to the body. It can be done, but it must be done carefully.

A Collaborative Solution to Finding the Proper Activity Level

As I stated above, there's no-one-size-fits-all solution to living the ideal active life with scoliosis. But I believe there's a specific solution for each individual patient. Everyone with scoliosis can benefit from an active life, and no one should be kept from the joys of physical activity.

The solution is to collaborate. Patients need to be tuned in to their bodies so they know what hurts and what doesn't. They also need to feel comfortable communicating how they feel to their parents, caregivers, loved ones, and especially the health-care professionals in their lives. Exercise and physical activity should be challenging, not painful. A doctor or qualified scoliosis chiropractor can help a patient determine the proper activity level, but it's vital that communication is honest and open. If a patient tries to tough things out or decides not to reveal an injury, it will only lead to setbacks and frustrations. But when patients, family members, medical professionals, and others operate with strong communication, patients benefit and progress is made.

The Ideal Lifestyle for Treating Scoliosis Effectively

People who want to make big changes in their lives often find success by examining and changing their lifestyles. In many cases where transformation is necessary, making small tweaks isn't enough to drive positive change.

For example, it's quite common for people to want to lose weight. Some people will go on diets for brief periods of time or begin exercise regimens. They notice some changes, but those changes rarely stick. They go back to their regular diets and normal routines and eventually find themselves right back where they started. It's a process that I think we're all familiar with, and it can be very frustrating.

When people succeed at changing themselves for the better, it's usually because they decide to make serious changes to their lifestyles. They don't go on diets; they change their diets permanently. They don't just join a gym; they make fitness an integral part of everyday living. It's not about quick fixes—it's all about developing new habits and entirely new routines.

For people with scoliosis, lifestyle can make a big difference when it comes to treating their condition effectively. Scoliosis is a condition that doesn't appear or disappear quickly. It develops slowly over time. Even cases that seem to have developed overnight have been progressing in the background. Likewise, reductions in abnormal spinal curvatures don't appear quickly or spontaneously. Rather, reductions take time and effort. That being the case, it's easy to see why small tweaks would not have the desired impact. Instead, changes should be made on a deeper, more holistic lifestyle level.

What Does the Word Lifestyle Mean?

Various sources provide different definitions of the word, but I would define it like this:

Lifestyle is the set of values, choices, attitudes, beliefs, opinions, motivations, needs, wants, and behaviors that determine a person's way of being. It's not so much about specific choices as it's about the fundamental aspects of a person's core that drive those choices. It's determined largely by each individual, but is greatly influenced by society, culture, family, and a person's economic realities. Lifestyle is also influenced heavily by a person's aspirations—it has a lot to do with how people see themselves in the present, but is also heavily impacted by people's notions of who they will *become*.

In terms of living with scoliosis, lifestyle is a serious consideration. The way a person approaches living will directly impact their ability to treat their condition. But scoliosis also presents limitations that contribute to a person's lifestyle.

Living with Scoliosis the Right Way

Scoliosis affects people from all backgrounds and walks of life. And it affects every individual differently. There's no single lifestyle that's appropriate for everyone who has scoliosis. But there are some lifestyle choices that can move patients in a positive direction:

- **Diet**—People who fuel themselves with balanced diets are more likely to respond favorably to treatment. Eliminating highly processed foods or those loaded with excess sugar in favor of whole, natural foods is an example of a lifestyle choice highly conducive to improved health for scoliosis patients.

- **Activity**—As I discussed in previous sections of this chapter, exercise and physical activity are key to living one's best life with scoliosis. Patients should understand that exercise isn't just something that can be done a few times. It needs to become a part of the daily routine. It shouldn't be seen as a passing fad; it needs to become part of one's lifestyle.

- **Social Life**—Humans are highly social creatures. Our lifestyles are determined largely by the people we spend the most time with. Therefore, if a scoliosis patient spends too much time with unhealthy or negative people, it will probably lead to them living an unhealthy, negative lifestyle. On the other hand, patients who socialize with positive, uplifting, and supportive people develop habits and lifestyle choices that are much more conducive to healing.

- **Mind-Set**—At the heart of everything is a person's mind-set. A person's lifestyle is cultivated initially in the mind. So if a person with scoliosis wants to change their lifestyle, it's critical to start with the space between the ears. A healthy, positive, open mind-set leads to better overall lifestyle choices. This is huge! So much so, that I will cover it in more detail in the next section.

What Is Your Scoliosis Lifestyle?

Whether you're a patient or parent, your lifestyle has a tremendous impact on the effects of scoliosis. If you recognize the need for change in order to cope with scoliosis more effectively, you may be interested in learning about tweaks or quick fixes. However, real change comes from deeper changes that happen on the lifestyle level. Obviously, changing one's tried-and-true, familiar lifestyle can be quite daunting and intimidating. But I can tell you that those who have done so successfully—and in the best interest of treating their scoliosis—are the ones who make the most progress.

The Healthy Scoliosis Mind-Set

In chapter 3, I discussed the power of a positive mental attitude and its ability to enhance the life—and treatment—of a scoliosis patient. I also brought up the idea of mind-set in the previous section on lifestyle. Mind-set is incredibly important when it comes to every aspect of scoliosis, so I thought it would be useful to dive back in to the topic here, in the context of overall health.

Perhaps there's no single type of mind-set that guarantees success with scoliosis, but there are certainly noticeable factors that seem to correspond to better outcomes for patients.

Once again, there are no one-size-fits-all solutions for those who have scoliosis. But I can offer some wisdom that can help patients and parents sharpen their mind-sets, toughen their ability to cope with the condition, and open them to new, more positive ways of thinking.

Belief, Acceptance, and Love

Scoliosis patients with healthy mind-sets don't fall into the trap of self-criticism or pity. Instead, they believe strongly in themselves as individuals. They accept themselves for who they are—not for who they would rather be—and they love themselves unconditionally. They even find a way to love their scoliosis! With this type of accepting mind-set, they're capable of achieving much more than the average person because they aren't weighed down by negative, critical self-talk. They're grateful to be here and honored by the opportunity to face the challenge of coping with scoliosis. This type of mind-set isn't the default reaction. It's normal for patients to turn to the negative view of things, but the ability to look at situations differently can be learned and ingrained through training.

Honesty and Purpose

People with healthy mind-sets spend time cultivating their ability to be honest—with themselves and others. They don't try to spin things in a positive light just to feel better or make others feel better. Instead, they're honest about how their condition makes them feel. This doesn't mean dwelling on the negative, though. It means recognizing that there are positive and negative aspects to all situations and scenarios. And when a person is honest about these things, it gives them the chance to live with genuine purpose. For scoliosis patients, purpose could mean finding a way to live the best life with the condition, or it might mean being driven by the promise of healing. Regardless, people with healthy mind-sets tend to develop this powerful combination of honesty and purpose better than most others.

Presence and Forward Movement

People with healthy mind-sets don't spend too much of their time lamenting the past or worrying about the future. They live their lives in the present moment, which means they don't miss out on what's happening in the here and now. Being present and mindful of the moment contributes to less strain and mental distress. It also helps people center their minds in a way that leads to greater openness, patience, and positivity. And when people are grounded in the present moment, they give themselves the best chance at moving forward in ways that are conducive to their values. For scoliosis patients, parents, and others who are affected by the condition, this creates a grounded, healthy mind-set.

Creating the Best Conditions for Healing Scoliosis

As a scoliosis chiropractor, I don't actually heal people's spines or reduce their curvatures. My patients are the ones doing the hard work and putting forth the effort. I'm simply guiding them. My job is to provide advice and expertise designed to create the best conditions for healing and reduction of curvatures.

By helping people condition themselves properly for success, I've guided countless individuals through the process of improving and reducing their spinal curvatures.

Basically, what you put into your body has a considerable impact on how it operates. This is why diet is so important for scoliosis patients. What a person reads and consumes, mentally, is also important for healing.

Output is also crucial. Especially when it comes to physical output. Working the body is a process that produces sweat—and a stronger, healthier body.

Diet, exercise, and lifestyle almost always come down to choices involving input and output. What are you putting into your body and mind? What are you producing and putting into the world? If these choices are healthy and lead to an improved body, mind, and world, it means conditions for the healing of scoliosis have been optimized. If not, then the path toward healing is a longer one.

What conditions are you creating with your choices? Are you doing everything you can to make healthy decisions, or are you sitting back and hoping for a miracle cure? The way you go about living your daily life will influence your ability to heal, particularly if you opt for chiropractic-centered treatment for scoliosis.

Hopefully I've convinced you of the importance of diet, exercise, and mind-set. Doing what you can to take care of yourself will help you handle scoliosis much more successfully, regardless of the treatment path you take.

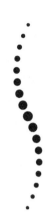

CHAPTER FIVE

Understanding the Facts About Scoliosis Treatment Options

IN THE PREVIOUS CHAPTERS of this book, I focused on the nature of scoliosis itself. I think it's important for people to fully understand the condition and how it affects people. I also feel that it's critical to understand that scoliosis affects many different kinds of people in many different ways.

Scoliosis, contrary to popular belief, is a highly treatable condition. But in order to understand how it can be treated effectively, patients and others should approach it with a comprehensive understanding of exactly what it means to have the condition.

In this chapter, I want to be very clear about the current landscape of scoliosis treatment options. Now that you have a fuller grasp on what it means to live with scoliosis and cope with it effectively, it's time to discuss what's possible. According to the status quo, watching and waiting—and hoping your scoliosis doesn't progress so you end up on the operating table—is the best treatment available for scoliosis. But I know that there's very little truth to that notion.

The reality is that scoliosis patients, their parents and their loved ones have an entire world of treatment options available to them. And in today's world, they don't need to be limited by geography. I speak to people all over the planet about scoliosis, and it's my hope that this book reaches even more people around the globe. What's more, my patients come to me from every time zone, every hemisphere, and every culture, seeking treatments that are more effective than those recommended by the medical establishment.

If you're dealing with scoliosis or you have a loved one who has the condition, this chapter will help guide you toward a path of treatment that provides hope, healing, and a more fulfilling life.

Five Key Questions to Ask before Treating Scoliosis

If you or a loved one has received a scoliosis diagnosis recently, you will probably be meeting doctors and other experts soon in order to begin the treatment process. You will probably find yourself doing a heavy amount of research as well, in order to determine the course of action that's most likely to produce the best solutions.

Because I'm an expert on scoliosis, patients, parents, and people just like you come to me seeking answers and advice on a daily basis. They're eager to learn more about the condition and what treatment might look like. They expect me to provide them with solid information, which I'm happy to do. But they don't always know what to ask.

If you're curious about next steps for scoliosis and want to prepare yourself with the right questions to ask—whether you're meeting with me or any other medical professional—it's critical that you ask the right questions. Otherwise, you may choose a treatment path that's not appropriate for you or your loved one.

There are numerous great questions to ask when you meet with a chiropractor or doctor regarding a scoliosis diagnosis. And each patient is different. The questions that are essential for one patient to ask may be different from those that are appropriate for another patient. That being said, I would like to highlight five key questions to ask before treating scoliosis.

The following questions will help you engage in a productive dialogue with your doctor or chiropractor that leads to the best possible treatment approach.

#1—"Is Scoliosis Your Primary Focus?"

For most doctors and chiropractors, scoliosis is one of a multitude of conditions that they diagnose and treat. They may be qualified to tell you that scoliosis is present and requires treatment. And they can perform a Cobb angle measurement. But if they aren't primarily focused on scoliosis, they may not be able to recommend the most beneficial approach to treatment.

#2—"What Types of Treatments Do You Employ?"

The majority of doctors take a single-minded approach to treating scoliosis. This approach involves observation, bracing, and surgery. They don't employ modalities such as exercise, physical therapy, or scoliosis-specific chiropractic care.

The best outcomes for scoliosis patients happen when a variety of treatment methods are used in conjunction with each other. For example, the Scoliosis Reduction Center combines scoliosis-specific chiropractic treatments with specialized physical therapy and exercise plans. Custom-designed braces are also employed using this treatment approach. This ensures that each treatment method works together with the others, and they build on one another. Approaching the condition from multiple angles increases the likelihood of reducing the abnormal curvature considerably. Therefore, it's critical that you assess the different approaches that a medical professional is capable of performing before moving ahead with treatment.

#3—"Have You Seen Cases Like This Before?"

This is a question I really wish more patients and parents would ask. The answer will reveal quite a bit about a doctor or chiropractor's level of expertise. Yes, every patient is unique, but your doctor or chiropractor should have a sense of the different ways in which scoliosis can manifest. If they have not seen a case like yours before, it could mean that they lack vital experience. If they *have* seen a case like yours, it's time to ask the next question.

#4—"What Was the Outcome When You Treated Similar Patients?"

Again, this question will reveal a lot of information about a doctor or chiropractor's ability to treat scoliosis effectively. If they can report improvements or reductions of abnormal curvatures when treating similar patients, that's great news! But if they can only report modest successes, or reveal that surgery was necessary in most cases, you should keep your treatment options open. I would also be wary of doctors or chiropractors who are unable to provide information regarding the success of their treatment approaches.

#5—"What Is the Goal of Your Treatment Approach?"

I'm surprised that this question doesn't get asked more often. But with so much on patients' and parents' minds, it's understandable. Different scoliosis experts have different goals in mind when they approach treating the condition. Some will move forward very conservatively, with a goal of using surgery once the curvature has progressed into severe territory. Others will make big claims about the goals they hope to achieve, but they will be unable to provide examples of success.

Consider this scenario: A patient receives advice from a surgeon on conservative treatment. From the surgeon's perspective, having a twenty-degree curve progress to a measurement of less than forty degrees would be considered a success in terms of keeping the patient from surgery. However, if the twenty-degree curve is managed from someone whose goal is to reduce it to ten degrees, it effectively creates a thirty-degree difference in results, even though "success" is achieved in both cases.

The goal of treatment here at the Scoliosis Reduction Center is to reduce abnormal spinal curvatures and help patients avoid surgery. Honestly, I think this should be the goal of any approach to treatment. Why? Because I know it's possible to achieve this goal more often than not. And I have patients from all around the world who can attest to our ability to achieve the goals of reduction and no surgery.

Does Your Child Need a Scoliosis Brace? Here's What You Need to Know

Adolescent idiopathic scoliosis affects millions of young people in the United States and all around the world. For many of those with the condition, life is altered in such a way that they're unable to participate in the types of activities that typically characterize adolescence. In most cases, treatment is passive, with doctors taking a wait-and-see approach, which, of course, yields no improvement. Eventually, these young people are fitted with braces, such as the Boston Brace.

Traditional braces have been used for decades to treat scoliosis among adolescents, but they're actually quite ineffective when it comes to actually reducing the curvature of the spine. At best, they may prevent further irregular curvature. Unfortunately, most of the time patients who are fitted with braces end up progressing to the point at which they require surgery to correct their condition, which is invasive and life-altering during a critical time in the life of an adolescent.

The Major Types of Scoliosis Braces

The traditional treatment of adolescent idiopathic scoliosis utilizes one of three main types of braces:

- Boston Brace
- Charleston Bending Brace (also known as the night-time brace)
- Milwaukee Brace

The Boston Brace

This brace, which is the most commonly used scoliosis brace in the United States, is a type of TLSO (Thoracic-Lumbo-Sacral-Orthosis) brace. It focuses on the mid to lower spine, and its purpose is to attempt to stabilize a lateral bending of a scoliosis curve. Developed in 1972 by doctors at the Boston Children's Hospital, this brace is typically constructed of hard, durable plastic, and wraps around the patient's rib cage, hips, and lower back beneath the arms.

The Boston Brace is mass-produced, which means that it's *not* custom designed for each patient. However, specialists use a number of methods and measures to ensure the proper fit and function. Even so, the person who fits the brace is likely someone who fits all kinds of prosthetics, not just scoliosis braces. Their goal is only to hold the spine from getting worse; the brace may "fit" the patient, but it may not be designed and optimized for reduction.

It's designed to be worn full time, which means that patients are directed to wear it eighteen to twenty-three hours a day, for up to five years. Eventually, patients should be weaned completely out of the brace. Under normal circumstances, Boston Braces are discontinued when a patient is close to skeletal maturity. This type of brace is rarely recommended for anyone past the point of growth because the goal of the apparatus is to simply hold the spine.

The idea behind this type of scoliosis brace is to squeeze or compress the irregular curvature of the spine in a manner that attempts to hold the spine from progressing any further. It uses specially placed pads to apply pressure to the curved areas of the spine. Meanwhile, a relief area of the brace is placed opposite the pad. Essentially, the pad squeezes the spine as part of what's known as a *three-point pressure system*.

The Boston Brace is meant to be uncomfortable by design. The idea is that the patient, through this discomfort, can attempt to stop the progression.

The Charleston Bending Brace

This brace is designed to be worn overnight during sleep. Developed in the late 1970s by doctors in Charleston, South Carolina, the idea behind this brace is to give those with adolescent idiopathic scoliosis the chance to reduce thoracolumbar curves during sleep. The doctors who developed the brace thought it could help patients avoid the stigma associated with wearing a full-time brace. They also attempted to take advantage of the non-weight-bearing postures common during sleep. The brace was designed in such a way to allow the pelvis to be manipulated and enhance the effect on some of the curves in the lower area of the spine.

The Charleston Bending Brace is molded in a manner that conforms to the patient's body while they're bent toward the outward bulge of their curve. It's meant to overcorrect the curvature. Due to this brace's design, it can't be worn in a standing position. It's limited to only sleeping. Many people question how effective a brace can be when it's only worn for a limited amount of time each day. I can understand the skepticism. What's more, this type of brace only addresses the bending associated with scoliosis. It does not address rotation.

Other nocturnal bracing apparatus similar to the Charleston Bending Brace include the Providence Brace and the Wilmington Brace.

The Milwaukee Brace

Also known as a CTLSO (Cervico-Thoraco-Lumbo-Sacral-Orthosis), the Milwaukee Brace is typically prescribed to treat high thoracic—mid-back—curves. Similar to the Boston Brace, this device features a bulkier design that extends all the way from the neck down to the pelvic region. The neck ring and pelvic girdle that comprise the brace are connected by metal bars that extend the torso's length and keep the head centered above the pelvis. Like the Boston Brace, this device uses strategically placed pads to squeeze the spine to try to stop progression.

The Milwaukee Brace has undergone a number of design improvements since its development by doctors at the Medical College of Wisconsin and Milwaukee Children's Hospital in the 1940s. The most commonly used design was established in 1975 and has remained virtually unchanged since then. The changes that *have* been implemented have been introduced in the interest of comfort. The results that are achieved are very similar to those of the Boston Brace because of the squeezing of the spine common to the operation of both apparatuses.

The Problems with Scoliosis Braces

You might think that because scoliosis braces are the most commonly used devices for treating the condition that they would be highly effective. Unfortunately, that just isn't the case.

These braces attempt to provide a two-dimensional solution for a three-dimensional condition. The Boston Brace, for example, has a small chance of preventing a curve from worsening, but due to its squeezing design, it can restrict and weaken the patient's spine and abdomen. Unfortunately, this can actually have an effect opposite of what's intended. Because it's designed to squeeze the spine without crucial strengthening and stabilizing, it can exacerbate the condition and weaken the spine. Additionally, there's a growing belief that the Boston Brace may even *increase* rigidity of the spine. Furthermore, due to this three-point pressure system, the Boston Brace applies pressure mostly from the side. It's believed that this can contribute to the worsening of rib deformities.

Patients who wear traditional scoliosis braces also cite a number of aspects that cause them inconvenience, pain and/or discomfort, including the following:

- restricted breathing
- sore or tight hip muscles
- red, raw, and sore skin
- heat-related discomfort
- restricted movement and an inability to bend the torso
- exercise difficulties

Furthermore, it's not uncommon for the devices like the Boston Brace and Milwaukee Brace to be fitted improperly, which leads to a number of serious side effects. Most notably, a brace that's too tight can lead to discomfort with breathing. Bowel obstructions can also occur when a scoliosis brace applies too much pressure against the ribs.

Another major concern with scoliosis braces is that they aren't worn according to prescription. Normally, this is because traditional braces typically become increasingly difficult to tolerate, which is a sign that the patient's curvature is progressing. Teenagers have enough to worry about without adding to their awkwardness with cumbersome scoliosis braces. Though there's the promise of a physical benefit, many teens weigh their options and conclude that the negative social aspects of wearing a brace aren't worth the potential physical relief they may experience. They're aware enough to notice that their abnormal posture and spinal curvature continue to progress in spite of the brace. So many of them decide that wearing a brace is just not worth it.

An Effective Alternative to Traditional Scoliosis Braces

At the Scoliosis Reduction Center, we take a proactive approach to the treatment of adolescent idiopathic scoliosis. We don't just wait and see; we get to work on our patients and provide them with the tools and techniques to strengthen their spines, improve function, and truly reduce their irregular curvatures. This approach is more natural, more functional, and involves a number of treatments that, when combined, provide relief and allow teens to experience their lives as fully as possible.

Yes, we use scoliosis bracing techniques and devices, but our methods involve pushing the spine in a corrective manner versus squeezing the spine in a way that limits function.

What Can a Scoliosis X-Ray Reveal about the Condition?

Contrary to popular belief, scoliosis is highly treatable. Here at the Scoliosis Reduction Center, we've seen patients transform their lives completely by taking part in our comprehensive treatment program. When patients approach their scoliosis with a positive attitude and a willingness to do what it takes to reduce their spinal curvatures, amazing things can happen. But before the first step of treatment can be taken, we need an accurate assessment and measurement. The gold standard today is the scoliosis X-ray.

Why Scoliosis X-Rays Are So Important

You might think that in the twenty-first century, a superior technology would exist. But the X-ray is still the most accurate, easily accessible, most cost-effective, and most reliable method of diagnosing and assessing scoliosis.

Certainly, there are other methods of screening for scoliosis. They just aren't as effective at identifying the condition. Or they're prohibitively expensive compared to the relative low cost of X-rays. For example, 3-D X-ray technology exists, but it's very expensive and time-consuming. Accurate scans also depend on the patient remaining perfectly still. Standing MRI scans are also used, but again, they're expensive and ultimately no more accurate than a scoliosis X-ray.

Obviously, X-rays provide two-dimensional imagery, while scoliosis is a three-dimensional condition. This means that it's critical to be able to interpret a scoliosis X-ray properly in order to provide patients with the best information and the most effective treatment plan.

Using 2-D Imagery for a 3-D Condition

There are limitations involved with using X-rays to diagnose, assess, and measure spinal curvature. Effective treatment of scoliosis requires a three-dimensional approach, and X-rays only provide a two-dimensional picture of what's happening with the spine.

However, experts who specialize in scoliosis understand how to use multiple X-rays to paint a complete picture of the spine.

Most doctors don't focus their practices strictly on scoliosis. They can tell patients that an abnormal curvature exists, and they can provide a scoliosis diagnosis based on what they see in an X-ray. But in most cases, they're unable to give patients accurate measurements. And because they lack the training and expertise to interpret scoliosis X-rays comprehensively, they're unable to give patients the proper recommendations.

Yes, it's easy to see the presence of an abnormal curvature, but measuring that curvature and providing the right advice for patients requires an expert's eye. Otherwise, different doctors who measure the same spine can produce wildly different measurements, which leaves patients in the dark when it comes to approaching their treatment properly.

It is, in fact, possible to use X-rays to evaluate scoliosis in a three-dimensional manner, but most doctors simply lack the proper know-how.

When patients come to me, I use multiple measurements to assess the condition. I also look at the spine from several different X-ray angles to measure twist, tilt, and other factors. There's more to measuring scoliosis than the Cobb angle. And devising the appropriate treatment plan is only possible when the condition is viewed from multiple angles.

The Right Way to Use Scoliosis X-Rays

Here at the Scoliosis Reduction Center, we use and refer to X-rays every day to treat our patients.

There are a few things that set us apart, though:

- We use the latest digital scoliosis X-ray technology, ensuring the greatest accuracy and the least exposure to radiation.
- We use small, specifically targeted X-rays to evaluate biomechanical integrity of the spine, which allows us to achieve more precise measurements.

- My focus is scoliosis. I've measured thousands of scoliosis X-rays—therefore, I have the ability to interpret a scoliosis X-ray more accurately than the average health-care practitioner. This gives me the ability to craft a much more effective treatment plan.

- Scoliosis X-rays are used at various points in the treatment process to measure progress, apply specific adjustments, prescribe exercises and ensure that the condition is targeted in the most efficient manner possible.

Concerns about Scoliosis X-Rays and Radiation

There are a lot of fears surrounding X-rays for scoliosis patients. For one thing, X-rays rarely reveal good news for scoliosis patients. But they also expose patients to a certain amount of radiation, which causes many patients to be reluctant about having X-rays taken.

I can understand why patients are discouraged by X-rays that increasingly show a progression of the spinal curvature. However, with the proper treatment, X-rays don't have to be bad news. Our patients receive the type of treatment that gets them to actually look *forward* to X-rays because they know they're likely to see improvement.

As for the radiation associated with a scoliosis X-ray, the risk is minimal, especially when images are taken using the most advanced, up-to-date digital technology.

Think about how digital cameras have revolutionized photography—they require less light and less exposure than their analog counterparts of the past. Today's X-ray equipment has advanced similarly. It releases very little radiation, and patients have nothing to fear about having multiple images taken.

The fact is that today's scoliosis X-rays emit about ten times less radiation than when I graduated from college twenty-two years ago. That's a huge reduction! And when you consider the minimal risks associated with X-rays against the consequences of not treating the condition properly, it's quite clear that the benefits outweigh the potential negatives by a massive margin.

Furthermore, I want patients to understand that we approach X-rays with the safety and health of our patients at the front of our minds. We use specially designed shielding to minimize the risk of radiation exposure. We also employ techniques like taking images from the back instead of the front, which reduces radiation exposure to the breasts and vital organs.

I understand why patients and parents may be concerned about radiation from scoliosis X-rays, but let me assure you that your health is our foremost focus!

Scoliosis X-Ray: Still the Gold Standard

A scoliosis X-ray is the best way to assess the condition and develop the proper treatment plan. It can reveal everything we need to know about an individual's specific curvature. Plus, it's inexpensive and easily accessible for patients regardless of location or circumstances.

The key is making sure the X-ray is interpreted properly by someone who knows scoliosis. When a scoliosis X-ray is performed by an expert and evaluated by someone who focuses on scoliosis, real change and improvement is possible.

What You Need to Know About Spinal-Fusion Scoliosis Surgery

Treating scoliosis with surgery is the default approach taken by the traditional medical establishment. It has become so normalized and so routine, though, that I'm afraid people don't fully understand what it means to undergo surgery for scoliosis.

Spinal-fusion scoliosis surgery, for example, is a serious procedure. It changes the body significantly, and it can alter the course of a patient's life irreversibly. Yes, surgery has become the standard for treatment; I just want patients and their families to understand what they're getting themselves into when they opt to engage in this approach.

Surgery has its place in the world of medicine, but it should never be seen as a cure for scoliosis. In my opinion, surgery should only be seen as a last resort. There are alternative, effective approaches to consider that are far less invasive—and considerably less expensive. Spinal-fusion scoliosis surgery is used so frequently that it has become routine, though. Patients and family members rarely question the conventional wisdom about surgery. And they almost never get the facts about surgery before opting to go under the knife.

Of course, I'm biased toward the chiropractic-centered approach to scoliosis treatment that we employ here at the Scoliosis Reduction Center. But I'm proud to stand behind the results we achieve every day with our patients. Patients often come to us feeling confused or scared by the prospect of impending surgery. They don't realize that there's another way. And they don't fully understand the consequences of watching and waiting on their way to the operating room.

We're able to give our patients a perspective that's rare in the world of scoliosis. And we're able to give them hope. If our treatment methods fail to produce results, surgery is always an option down the road. I just think it's important for patients to understand exactly what spinal-fusion scoliosis surgery entails.

Here's what you should know:

Spinal-Fusion Surgery Is Not a Scoliosis Cure

Can spinal-fusion scoliosis surgery make a spine straighter? Yes. Is spinal-fusion scoliosis surgery a cure? No!

To be perfectly honest, there's no cure for scoliosis. No single procedure or form of therapy will ever magically cause the condition to disappear, and there's no pill for scoliosis patients to take that will reverse their spinal curvatures.

Spinal-fusion surgery can absolutely reduce or stabilize a curve. It does not, however, return the body to a normal state. It does not address any of the underlying causes of the condition. In fact, it can introduce a whole new slate of potential problems. What's more, patients can experience a worsening of their condition even after they have undergone "successful" spinal-fusion scoliosis surgery!

Spinal-Fusion Surgery Involves the Removal of Discs

Spinal discs are crucial to the human anatomy. But they're technically not essential for having a functional body. One sometimes overlooked aspect of spinal-fusion surgery is the fact that it involves the removal of these discs, as if they're merely accessories.

For many patients, the removal of spinal discs will not create a noticeable impact. But for others, the loss of these shock-absorbing components of the spine contributes to further damage, particularly if they're subject to traumatic forces. Automobile accidents, for instance, can introduce trauma and shock, with forces transferred to rigid surgical rods. This can cause an incredible amount of damage to the body.

Spinal-Fusion Surgery Can Reduce Mobility Considerably

Scoliosis surgery has become so normalized in our culture that patients believe they can go on living and moving their bodies just as they did prior to surgery. While it's true that some patients can experience similar levels of mobility before and after surgery, this is rare. In most cases, patients experience a noticeable *decrease* in mobility.

According to one study, mobility decreases by an average of 25 percent after spinal-fusion scoliosis surgery (Spine, 2006). Another study revealed that decreases in mobility remain even after twenty years (Spine, 2006). I've seen countless patients over the years, and it's clear to me that patients who undergo surgery suffer a marked decrease in mobility compared to their counterparts who undergo proper forms of treatment.

Far too many scoliosis patients opt to undergo surgery without realizing the permanent effects it can have on the body's mobility. I think it's critical to reckon with this reality before making such a significant decision.

Spinal-Fusion Surgery Should Not Be Performed on Growing Bodies

When Harrington rods are installed inside patients with bodies that are still growing, the results can be extremely problematic. Abnormal curvatures can persist and continue to develop above and below the fused areas of the spine. It's also possible for patients to outgrow the rods. When this happens, secondary surgeries become necessary in order to remove and replace the original rods. This is complicated, expensive, and likely to introduce further complications.

Of course, this ties in to the watch-and-wait approach. Surgeons are wisely unwilling to operate on patients whose bodies continue to grow and develop. But instead of offering proactive alternatives to treatment, traditional doctors and orthopedic specialists recommend a strategy of observation and traditional squeezing bracing, which typically only ensures that scoliosis will continue to develop. Inevitably, this approach leads to surgery later in life, once the body has stopped growing.

Alternative Treatments Can Improve Surgical Outcomes for Scoliosis Patients

There's no harm in treating scoliosis with alternative methods that combine chiropractic care and scoliosis-specific physical therapy. These types of treatments aren't invasive, nor do they produce irreversible negative results. When properly administered, they have the potential to reduce abnormal curvatures, as well as improve key quality-of-life indicators such as pain and sleep patterns. Most importantly, these types of treatments can produce results that ensure surgery remains a last resort.

But let's say surgery truly is inevitable. If surgery absolutely must happen, alternative treatment methods can benefit patients considerably. Chiropractic-centered treatments strengthen the spine and give it increased flexibility. This can help ensure greater success—and fewer complications—in surgery.

The bottom line is that spinal-fusion scoliosis surgery does not have to be seen as inevitable. Alternative treatment methods, like those we employ here at the Scoliosis Reduction Center, provide relief and results. Our approach puts patients in the driver's seat, and it allows them the opportunity to make a better life for themselves without surgery. But if for some reason surgery is still required, those patients are much more likely to experience positive results if they engage in chiropractic-centered treatment. To me, that's the perfect win-win scenario.

What Happens after Scoliosis Surgery?

Perhaps this is an oversimplification, but typically, there are two paths a person can take once they've received a scoliosis diagnosis. One is the path of traditional treatment. It involves watching and waiting—and not much active involvement from the patient. Eventually, this path can lead to surgery.

The other path involves a less traditional approach, often guided by someone like me, a scoliosis-focused chiropractor. This path requires patients to take a more active approach to their healing, and it leads *away* from surgery.

I can understand why the traditional path is so heavily traveled. In our society, we tend to look for quick fixes, magic pills and fixes that don't involve changes in behavior or lifestyle. To many scoliosis patients, surgery is a promise that helps them see a more hopeful future, so they follow orders from their doctors and patiently wait for the day they can finally go under the knife. They're convinced that the path they travel is the only one that leads to relief. And because the medical establishment endorses this path, they have no reason to look elsewhere for alternative approaches to treatment.

Unfortunately, scoliosis patients don't always travel this path with a full understanding of what it means.

The Realities of Scoliosis Surgery

Spinal-fusion surgery for scoliosis is far from a fix for the condition. However, it may stabilize the spine and halt the progression of an abnormal spinal curvature. It's costly and invasive, but for many patients, the promise of relief is well worth the price they pay financially.

Individuals with scoliosis want relief so badly that they may not recognize the hardships that can come with surgery. And if they have been informed of alternative treatment approaches, such as the chiropractic-centered model, they may be intimidated by the sheer amount of work and participation that's required of them. Or they have been convinced by medical professionals that alternative approaches are simply not legitimate.

Regardless, I think it's important for patients to understand what surgery truly entails.

Basically, most scoliosis surgeries involve the use of hooks and screws that are attached to the spine. These fasteners are used to anchor long rods. The surgeon will use the rods to reposition critical areas of the spine, reducing lateral curvatures.

Additionally, surgeons will graft bone to the segments of the vertebrae that will be fused.

This is a serious procedure. But what I just described is only the beginning. What happens *after* scoliosis surgery is important to understand as well.

Life after Scoliosis Surgery

The rods that are installed during surgery act as splints to hold the spine in position while the fusion process occurs. This can take up to six months, with fusion continuing for up to a full year. Once the fusion process has completed, the spine is kept from curving abnormally by the recently fused bone. The rods typically remain in the body because removing them would require an additional surgery!

As for the patient's ability to live a normal life, it's crucial to understand that recovery takes time.

A patient will be allowed to return home after surgery, but they will be weak, medicated, and in need of time to rest. Bending, lifting, twisting, driving, and numerous other activities are forbidden during the initial few weeks after surgery. Moreover, patients will require assistance from a friend, family member, or other loved one to keep up with daily care and tasks.

Pain management is also a serious consideration after scoliosis surgery. Often, patients will be prescribed narcotics, which will ease their pain and discomfort. However, these drugs will also limit cognitive ability and reduce overall energy levels significantly.

Patients and their caregivers also need to be diligent in the care of the surgical incision site. It needs to be kept clean and dry to ensure the best possible recovery. Showers can be taken, but the incision site must be covered, either with a dressing provided by the surgeon's staff or with common kitchen plastic wrap.

After about two weeks, the patient will meet with their doctor for a follow-up appointment. This gives the patient the opportunity to ask questions and report on how they're feeling. It gives the surgeon the opportunity to assess the patient and collaborate on a plan to move forward.

After the First Follow-Up and Beyond

Patients are understandably anxious to get back to normal life at this point, but serious precautions still need to be made. Patients will be able to engage in social activities, ride in vehicles, go back to school, and transition away from narcotic pain relief. However, rest and recovery should remain the top priorities.

X-rays are taken at about the six-week mark following surgery. At this time, if the spine is healing properly, surgeons will permit patients to drive again and resume more normal activity.

Between six and twelve months after surgery, the fusion process will reach completion, and the patient will be able to resume most normal activities. But full and complete recovery does not occur until after the patient has healed from any trauma related to their surgery. This can take up to two years. But in reality, surgical patients are never really fully recovered—surgery is serious, and it impacts the way a person lives their life, even if the surgery is successful at stabilizing an abnormally curved spine.

Obviously, every patient is different, but this timeline is quite typical for those who travel the path of scoliosis treatment that leads to surgery.

The Chiropractic-Centered Treatment Path for Scoliosis

The path of healing I advocate for is much different. There's no watching and waiting to see what happens; we get to work. Through the efforts of the patient, my staff, and myself, spinal curvatures can be reduced. It's not an easy process for patients to endure, but in my opinion, it's far preferable to surgery. My goal is to help patients avoid surgery. Conventional wisdom may say that surgery is the best we can do for scoliosis. But I believe otherwise, and my patients can prove it!

Scoliosis Treatment: What Is the Cost?

Throughout this book, I've written about numerous aspects of scoliosis treatment. I've spent a lot of time comparing and contrasting the traditional, surgery-focused approach with the chiropractic-centered approach with the hope of convincing readers like you of the benefits of engaging in alternative treatments. At this point in your research into the condition, you're probably wondering, "What's the cost of scoliosis treatment?"

Regardless of the treatment path chosen, the costs involved can be alarming. In order to receive *any* kind of treatment, a significant financial commitment must be made. That's why I think it's so important to look at the cost of treatment in terms of value.

The Cost of Traditional Scoliosis Treatment

First, let's take a look at the costs associated with treating mild scoliosis in the traditional model.

Monitoring a mild curve for just one year, which includes doctor visits, exams, and X-rays can cost between $3,000 and

$4,000, typically. This means that patients are paying thousands of dollars every single year to simply watch and wait. Observation is the standard of traditional treatment, but it actually does nothing to treat the condition! To me, this does not represent a good value at all.

What about moderate scoliosis?

At this stage of traditional treatment, traditional bracing enters the picture. Costs can vary, but generally fall in the $5,000–$10,000 range for the apparatus itself. The costs associated with doctors fitting the brace add even more to the cost, meaning that moderate scoliosis costs the average patient more than $10,000 each year. And this is on top of the costs associated with observation.

Yes, this is a lot of money. But moderate scoliosis becomes even more costly when you consider the value patients receive for their treatment. With traditional bracing and observation to treat moderate scoliosis, patients can hope to—at best—stabilize the spine and prevent further progression. In most cases, however, these traditional braces do little more than slow down the progression of the curvature slightly. They're also incredibly cumbersome and make normal life more difficult to live. I don't think this is a good value, personally.

Now let's talk about severe scoliosis.

Severe scoliosis is ultimately treated through spinal-fusion surgery, which typically costs at least $100,000. In many cases, the cost of surgery reaches $150,000 or even more. And that's in addition to costs associated with X-rays, doctor visits, bracing, and other procedures, not to mention costs associated with complications or subsequent surgeries later in life.

Surgery is also invasive, and isn't guaranteed to fix the scoliosis. Considering the high cost of surgery, does it seem like a good value to you? It certainly doesn't seem like one to me!

The Cost of Chiropractic-Centered Treatment for Scoliosis

The costs of treating scoliosis using the chiropractic-centered treatment approach aren't insignificant, but when you look at the differences between alternative treatments and traditional ones, it's obvious that the chiropractic approach provides a better value.

Think about what you would do if you had $200,000 to spend on scoliosis treatment. Would you spend it on treatment that leads to further progression and, eventually, invasive surgery that's not guaranteed to provide relief? Or would you invest in regular treatments from someone who uses an approach that's been shown to actually reduce spinal curvatures? No matter what, you're going to invest a large amount of money. But it seems quite clear to me that the best value in scoliosis treatment lies with the chiropractic-centered approach that my team and I use here at the Scoliosis Reduction Center.

What Can Go Wrong while You're Watching and Waiting with Scoliosis?

By now, I hope I've laid out the differences between traditional and chiropractic-centered scoliosis treatments in a manner that makes the distinctions between the two approaches clear to you.

Essentially, the traditional approach is one that tells patients, "Sorry. There's nothing we can do."

The chiropractic-centered approach, on the other hand, tells patients, "Let's get to work treating your scoliosis!" This may be an oversimplification, but it's not far from the truth.

The reality is that the traditional approach to treating scoliosis is characterized by ongoing observation instead of decisive action. Observation isn't a bad thing, necessarily. In fact, I would agree that it's critical to keep an eye on the spine to determine how well it responds to treatment. But when watching and waiting becomes the primary focus of treatment, scoliosis can only get worse over time.

Don't Ignore the Check-Engine Light!

If you own a car, you know exactly what I'm referring to here!

A lot of people will notice that their check-engine light becomes activated on their dashboard, or they notice that their vehicle has begun to make a strange sound, but they fail to do anything about it. They continue driving the car, watching and waiting until they can no longer ignore what might be going wrong under the hood. Some of them even go to great lengths to turn off the light while ignoring the underlying problem. *Out of sight, out of mind*, they think.

Eventually, these auto owners will run into situations that require them to seek intervention from an expert. More often than not, they find that they let a minor, inexpensive problem become a major, costly one because they decided to watch and wait instead of taking action.

To me, this isn't unlike the traditional approach to treating scoliosis. The body produces a number of signs and symptoms that reveal something is amiss. A diagnosis is made, but action isn't taken. Instead, the watching and waiting approach is prescribed. This leads to further progression of the abnormal curvature, which in turn can lead to expensive, invasive surgery.

What Can Happen while You Wait with Scoliosis?

Watching and waiting, while not likely to introduce unusual or unexpected complications, does nothing to correct abnormal spinal curvatures. Observation only leads to further progression, and ensures a greater likelihood of surgery becoming the only remaining option for treatment.

While patients watch and wait, they miss out on the opportunity to take a proactive approach to treatment that can not only stabilize curvatures, but also actually reduce them. They miss out on the benefits of things like scoliosis-specific exercises, physical therapy, and chiropractic care. For adolescents, watching and waiting means being sentenced to a traditional, cumbersome squeezing brace, which can harm their ability to get the most out of their teen years.

Watching and waiting isn't a strategy for success, in my opinion. It's little more than a strategy that increases the likelihood of patients walking the path that leads to surgery.

My goal with my practice is to do the exact opposite—I'm successful when I help patients *avoid* surgery! The contrast couldn't be starker.

If you're a scoliosis patient, or you're the parent of a child with scoliosis, I can understand why you may be convinced that watching and waiting is your best course of action. But I urge you to consider alternative forms of treatment. Otherwise, your watching and waiting could have you or your child missing out on the best things in life.

What Scoliosis Treatment Approach Is Right for You?

I've explained the contrasts between the traditional approach to scoliosis treatment and chiropractic-centered approach throughout this chapter, and I hope I've made the distinctions as clear as possible for you.

Making decisions regarding health care is a serious process. It shouldn't be taken lightly. Patients, parents, and others who may be touched by scoliosis want to make the best decisions, but they need to do so with the best possible information. There are countless books, articles, blog posts, and journals that describe the traditional, surgery-focused approach. Unfortunately, the literature pertaining to the chiropractic-centered approach isn't as easy to locate. That is why I think this chapter is so important.

I'm obviously biased toward the approach I employ, but that's because I believe in it so strongly—and I've seen firsthand what it can do for people whose lives are impacted by scoliosis. You should make your decisions regarding treatment carefully, and you should listen to a variety of voices. I just hope that mine is one of them, and that you hear the promise of my message.

In the following chapter, I will take my message even further as I break down the approach that I've seen work so well for so many people.

CHAPTER SIX

Chiropractic-Centered Scoliosis Treatment and the Patient-Focused Approach

NOW THAT I'VE COVERED the facts about scoliosis treatment approaches, it's time to dive into the topic I'm most passionate about—the chiropractic-centered approach to scoliosis treatment. This is at the heart of my practice, and it's the reason why patients from all around the world seek out the Scoliosis Reduction Center. My approach is different than the traditional model in many important ways, some of which I've highlighted in previous chapters and sections of this book.

Because the chiropractic-centered approach is relatively modern and misunderstood, I feel it's important to discuss the facts about it while debunking some of the myths. Also, I want to talk about some key differences between the traditional model of treatment and the one I believe in. For example, did you know that there are major differences between traditional scoliosis braces and the braces we use here at the Scoliosis Reduction Center?

The key to this approach is the fact that it's centered and focused on the patient. You may be wondering why that's notable—after all, isn't all medicine patient-centered? Well, the truth is that traditional treatment paths place the patient nearer to the margins than the center of the action, and I think that's a huge mistake.

There are reasons to believe in the traditional approach and its ability to help patients. But I don't think those reasons are rooted in as much reality as the establishment might have you believe. Furthermore, I truly think the reasons for taking the chiropractic-centered approach to scoliosis treatment are far more compelling—and more rooted in the reality of what it means to have scoliosis while trying to live a rich, fulfilling life.

Let's begin by taking a look at some of the reasons why traditional treatment options leave so much to be desired. Then, I will get into the heart of why I believe the chiropractic-centered approach is the right one for a new, better way of dealing with scoliosis.

Three Reasons Why Traditional Scoliosis Treatment Falls Short

As I alluded to in the previous chapter, it's relatively easy to find information about the traditional model of scoliosis treatment. This approach has been ingrained into the conventional wisdom regarding the condition, and is usually taken at face value without any skepticism. It's not so easy to find information that describes the ways in which the traditional approach falls short.

In this section, I want to shed more light on the traditional treatment approach to scoliosis. It's important for me to offer my perspective as a scoliosis chiropractor in order to ensure that patients and parents have the best information available to make decisions regarding treatment. Please note that it isn't my intention to cast doubt on the reputations of the many medical professionals who treat scoliosis using the traditional model. Rather, I think it's important to inform you and other readers of the areas where the traditional approach may not be as promising as many people would have you believe.

#1—Surgery Is Never Guaranteed to Positively Alter Scoliosis Signs or Symptoms

The centerpiece of the traditional approach to scoliosis treatment is surgery. Patients go through months—if not years or decades—of patient observation until they're told their scoliosis is severe enough to warrant surgery. It may seem backward, but the diagnosis of severe scoliosis is a triumph for many patients because it means they can finally go under the knife.

I understand why scheduling a surgery for scoliosis would seem like a relief. But I think it's crucial to consider the fact that there's no evidence that symptoms and signs can be altered through spinal-fusion surgery in the long term (Scoliosis, 2008). What's more, a number of complications can arise that introduce problems that would not have been experienced otherwise.

#2—Traditional Scoliosis Bracing Comes with Some Unwelcome Side Effects

When a teen is fitted with a traditional scoliosis brace such as the well-known Milwaukee or Boston Brace, the process is undertaken with a great deal of hope. Bracing, they're told, will help them stabilize their spines so they can live more normal, active lives, eventually. Sadly, patients aren't always informed of the negative side effects that can come with scoliosis bracing.

Due to the three-point pressure system (squeezing) that these braces use, they actually make the rib deformity worse!

First of all, traditional braces must be worn for at least sixteen hours a day, if not longer. Secondly, traditional scoliosis braces have been linked to incidences of depression, low self-esteem, and reduced quality of life for those who are fitted with them. Finally, teens who wear traditional scoliosis braces experience isolation and social anxiety at high rates compared to their peers.

And that's not all—traditional braces can actually decrease spinal flexibility, which only accelerates the "need" for expensive and invasive surgical procedures. And due to the squeezing three-point pressure system used by traditional braces, any rib deformities that are present can actually be made worse!

#3—Restrictions and Limitations Keep People from Doing What They Love

Young people with mild scoliosis may have symptoms that make the condition noticeable, but they're typically able to participate in life in a manner that allows them to explore their favorite passions and pursuits. Scoliosis does not keep them from doing what they love, and yet they and their parents often seek advice from traditional doctors regarding the condition. In most cases, they're advised to wait and see what happens.

Typically, a patient will receive a diagnosis of mild scoliosis and then be told to return to the doctor about six months later for more X-rays. Because young people's bodies can grow and change so quickly, that small, six-month window is enough time to allow the scoliosis to progress quickly into moderate or even severe territory. When curvatures progress quickly through watching and waiting, doctors will typically place restrictions on their young patients, which deteriorates their quality of life. Teens are told not to participate in certain sports or physical activities, and that can deflate the mood of the average adolescent completely.

And because of the progressive nature of scoliosis, those restrictions are almost never lifted. Instead, the scoliosis continues to progress to the point where, eventually, surgery is recommended to stabilize it.

Scoliosis Treatment Doesn't Have to Be Like This

These are just three reasons why traditional treatment falls short, but I could come up with even more. The point is that traditional treatment isn't always what it's cracked up to be. Yes, it may provide relief, but the road to relief winds through some very difficult terrain.

Chiropractic-centered treatment is much different. It's proactive and patient-centered. It's designed to help patients avoid surgery and get back to doing what they love. It's far from a magic, miracle solution for scoliosis, but I believe it can be far more effective than traditional treatments can be.

Treating Scoliosis—Five Reasons Why Watching and Waiting Won't Work

Initially, the traditional approach to treating scoliosis is conservative and seemingly sensible. Experts in the realm of conventional treatment agree that the best approach is to watch and wait. They err on the side of being reactive instead of proactive, and they convince patients and their families that their methods are practical, rational, and grounded in the most modern best practices. But all the watching and waiting that's done by scoliosis patients never improves the condition. In most cases, watching and waiting means watching as a spinal curvature progresses, and then, depending on the amount of progression, waiting to undergo expensive and invasive surgery.

Fortunately, alternative approaches to scoliosis treatment are gaining credibility and popularity. Here at the Scoliosis Reduction Center, we take a decidedly proactive approach to treating the condition. And we see people every single day for whom the traditional, watch-and-wait method is just not good enough.

With our chiropractic-centered treatment, patients feel like they're in the driver's seat. They're encouraged to be active and to engage in treatments that actually reduce spinal curvatures and help them avoid surgery. Our results speak for themselves— patients not only find relief for the physical aspects of scoliosis, but also find that our approach allows them to feel a significant mental and emotional boost. Instead of watching and waiting, they're taking charge of their condition and engaging in treatment that gives them the chance to live their best lives.

And yet the traditional watch-and-wait approach continues to reign supreme.

If you or your child are dealing with a scoliosis diagnosis, you may feel like you're stuck between a rock and a hard place. On one hand, you have the experts who recommend the watch-and-wait approach to treatment. On the other hand, you feel a need to be more proactive with the condition, which is what the experts seem to discourage.

Watching and waiting seems sensible, and it has the backing of orthopedic surgeons and other experts. But there's a lot those experts won't tell you.

Here are five reasons why watching and waiting won't work when it comes to treating scoliosis:

#1—It Does Not Stop the Progression of Abnormal Spinal Curvatures

I can't be more explicit about this. Watching and waiting is simply not a healing strategy. The fact is that this approach will more than likely not yield positive results. The nature of untreated scoliosis is to continue its progression. So when you fail to be proactive in treatment, the condition is allowed to continue progressing over time.

And guess what? Eventually, it will progress to the point where surgery presents itself as the only viable option for relief. And even then, surgery isn't guaranteed to stop the progression of the curvature, much less reverse it. But it *is* guaranteed to cost a lot of money.

#2—It Leaves Patients and Family Members Feeling Powerless

Most people, when faced with a challenge or a medical diagnosis, feel compelled to do something to overcome it. And for most conditions or illnesses, patients and their families are empowered with options and potential actions. When your child scrapes their knee or suffers a playground injury, there's no watching and waiting! You take action and participate in the healing of the condition. But when it comes to scoliosis treatment, watching and waiting is presented as the best option in many cases. This leaves patients and family members feeling as if they have no agency or ability to take action. Instead, they must bide their time and pray for an unprecedented improvement.

#3—It Represents a Huge Missed Opportunity

When a patient is told to wait six months after their diagnosis to come back for another examination, that's six months during which they could be actively addressing their condition. Instead, they're directed to sit still and watch the days on the calendar float by. In many cases, when they come back to the doctor, their curve has progressed. At this point, discussion of next steps involves more invasive treatment and, possibly, surgery.

All the time spent watching and waiting could have been used as an opportunity to address the condition directly through a chiropractic-centered treatment program. Treatment is most effective when curves are less severe. Smaller curvatures are much more manageable, and potential outcomes are far more favorable when the condition is treated as early as possible.

#4—It Almost Always Leads to Surgery

Sooner or later, watching and waiting draws patients and their families to a single solution—surgery. Of course, surgeons see surgery as the most effective solution because that's their specialty. Unfortunately, not all surgeons are up to speed on what can be done proactively for scoliosis. It reminds me of the old saying, "When your only tool is a hammer, every problem looks like a nail."

What's more, surgery can't be considered a cure for the condition. Yes, it may stabilize the spine and prevent continued progression, but it does nothing to address the underlying cause or causes of scoliosis. It can also introduce new problems. For example, spinal-fusion surgery involves the removal of spinal discs that are responsible for cushioning the spine from impact. Without them, the body (and the surgically implanted rods) must absorb shock and impact, leading to further potential complications and injury.

Note that sometimes adolescent cases don't progress to the point where surgery is recommended. These patients are told to continue watching and waiting into adulthood while their curves continue progressing slowly. Eventually, the curvatures reach the surgical level, but surgeons may not want to proceed with surgery because of the increased risk level associated with adult surgery.

#5—It Can Make Patients and Family Members Feel Hopeless

Hope may be an intangible quality that's impossible to measure, but it's incredibly powerful when facing an illness or a condition like scoliosis. Hope is what gets people through their toughest times, and it can have a considerable impact on overall well-being.

However, when patients and parents are told to watch and wait for a curvature progression to reach a certain level so surgery can be performed, it removes hope from the equation entirely.

Hope is essential for healing, but it gets pushed to the margins when taking the watch-and-wait approach to scoliosis treatment. Thankfully, you don't have to just bide your time and observe. You can be hopeful, and you can be proactive. Our approach here at the Scoliosis Reduction Center builds confidence, creates measurable improvements, helps patients avoid surgery and, importantly, restores hope.

Patient-Centered Scoliosis Treatment—What Does It Mean?

In the beginning of this chapter, I introduced the concept of patient-centered scoliosis treatment. In my opinion, keeping the patient at the center of focus should be the goal of any practitioner. Unfortunately, in our modern medical landscape, the patient has been pushed to the sidelines in nearly all aspects of care. This has become so widespread that people consider it normal to feel like they're on the outside looking in at their own treatment!

As it turns out, the approach that puts the patient front and center is becoming increasingly rare. Medicine is big business in our culture. When dollar signs are involved, patients turn into little more than contributors to a system that's designed to extract

SCOLIOSIS HOPE

as much money as possible from their wallets. Patient preferences and values have become unimportant to many health-care providers, and their opinions are taken into account less and less as time goes on.

The patient-centered approach I take to treating scoliosis is different. In my opinion, it's one of the things that sets me apart from those who practice typical health care, not to mention scoliosis-specific care.

But what does the patient-centered approach mean to me as a scoliosis chiropractor?

Patients Deserve to Be Comfortable

One of the tenets of patient-centered care is that patients ought to be comfortable with the treatment they receive. Their physical comfort is important, but so is their mental and emotional comfort. They should understand their treatments completely and never feel ill at ease about receiving them.

A Patient's Values and Preferences Should Be Respected

Decisions regarding care and treatment should be made in collaboration with the patient. It's also important to understand that patients are human beings with meaningful values and preferences. As such, they should be treated with respect and dignity.

Patients Should Be at the Center of Integration and Coordination of Care

As long as a patient is able to make sound decisions, they should be considered the focus of integration and coordination of care. In the case of adolescents and younger children, parents should also have a primary role in the leadership of the treatment approach and how it's managed. Patients and parents shouldn't

190

be left to wonder what's next or how certain aspects of care work alongside others.

Patients Should Be Educated and Informed

In many medical situations, patients are kept in the dark when it comes to the reality of their condition. This leads to anxiety, stress and a belief that whatever is happening to them is completely out of their control. I believe that patients need to be informed and educated as to the true nature of their condition and their ability to overcome it.

Patients Deserve to Involve Family, Friends, and Loved Ones in Their Care

I'm often amazed by what my patients are capable of doing during their treatment. But I'm even more amazed by how much support they receive from family members, friends, and other loved ones. There's a strong correlation between the support of others and a patient's ability to undergo treatment successfully, so it's critical to ensure the involvement of people who can serve to aid the healing process. Denying these crucial connections only serves to prolong treatment, decrease morale, and make patients feel isolated.

Patient-Centered Care and the Chiropractic-Centered Approach Go Hand in Hand

A chiropractic mind-set is at the center of my approach to treating scoliosis, and patients are always at the center of my attention when it comes to the reasons why I do what I do. I'm motivated by a desire to help people live full lives that are not limited by scoliosis, which means that I'm only successful when I put patients first. The reason I became a scoliosis chiropractor is because I realized scoliosis-centered chiropractic care is the best way to treat scoliosis successfully. It's an approach that puts patients at the center of their own care, which is one of the primary reasons it's so successful.

It may seem like patient-centered care is going out of style these days, but rest assured, I will always consider the patient to be the primary focus of my practice.

A New Brace for a New Era of Scoliosis Correction

Previously in this book, I discussed the facts about treating scoliosis in young people using traditional, TLSO (Thoraco-Lumbar Sacral Orthosis) bracing apparatus. Devices like the Boston Brace, Milwaukee Brace, or the Charleston Bending Brace were once seen as major innovations in the world of scoliosis treatment, and they still have their place today. However, these braces are far from the being on the cutting edge of modern scoliosis correction technology.

Traditional braces like these continue to use designs from decades ago, and few innovations have been introduced in the last forty or fifty years. Yes, they can be effective in the best-case scenario at holding the spine from progressing, but more often than not, they serve as clunky and cumbersome reminders of a condition that has serious impacts on how young people live their lives.

More importantly, traditional scoliosis braces can only promise to stop or slow the progression of an abnormal curvature. Even when they're worn for sixteen or more hours each day for years, they have little effect on reducing an abnormal curve.

I know there's a better way to approach scoliosis bracing—one that actually improves the condition, reduces curvatures, and helps restore function.

Scoliosis Correction in 3-D

If you have been reading my blog or have heard me speak, you know that I like to describe scoliosis as a 3-D condition. To me, it's not possible to treat scoliosis effectively as a two-dimensional condition, and yet that's the approach used by virtually every conventional treatment method.

The fact is that scoliosis is highly complex, and reducing it to two dimensions (i.e. left to right, forward to backward, etc.) ignores most of the picture. It's a lot like the difference between looking at a postcard of the beach and experiencing the setting in real life. The postcard can give you a sense of reality, but it's severely limited and is nothing more than a mere snapshot.

Traditional, TLSO bracing techniques treat scoliosis in a two-dimensional manner, which is why they aren't nearly as effective as more modern methods. Fortunately, new approaches exist. The ScoliBrace®, for example, uses a 3-D approach, and when it's implemented alongside chiropractic care, exercise, and therapy, it can actually reduce curvatures dramatically and make corrections to the condition.

What Makes ScoliBrace® Different?

The ScoliBrace® offers a number of advantages over traditional scoliosis braces:

- It uses the most effective corrective principles of the traditional, TLSO braces without including the problematic aspects of them.
- It is overcorrective, or as I like to say, *supercorrective*, which means that it positions the spine in an opposite mirror image of how the scoliosis is shaped within an individual's body. This allows for the reduction of curvatures in a majority of cases, in addition to improvements in

shoulder level, rib humping, and the body's overall aesthetic appearance.

- It is used in conjunction with BraceScan 3-D imaging software, which allows for a custom fit designed specifically for each individual patient.

- In addition to BraceScan technology, the ScoliBrace® is created with input from X-rays and posture photos, and is custom designed for each patient using CAD (computer-aided design) software

- It is designed to integrate more comfortably into a patient's life—opening and closing the brace happens at the front of the device, making it easier to wear and remove without requiring extra assistance. What's more, the ScoliBrace® is available in a variety of colors and patterns, which gives patients the chance to personalize the device as they see fit.

- Although individual results vary, it can reduce curvatures, reduce pain, improve posture, and enhance cosmetic aspects

ScoliBrace®: Part of a Comprehensive Approach to Scoliosis Correction

When I see young patients and talk to their families, I sense a great deal of frustration with the traditional scoliosis treatment approach. Adolescents are in the midst of a time in their lives when they should be looking to the future and dreaming of possibilities. Life should seem limitless to them. Unfortunately, the traditional treatment approach is all about limitations.

Traditional external bracing methods are designed to limit movement and limit the progression of the spine's abnormal curvature. They're designed to squeeze the spine instead of push it. These braces also limit the ways a young person can go about living life. They put patients on a path that often leads to surgery, which is a sort of internal bracing that may be very limited in its ability to improve the lives of scoliosis patients.

When I was younger, I felt limited by debilitating migraines. Later in life when I became a chiropractor, I felt limited by the idea that I could only manage—and not improve—conditions like scoliosis. I found a better way to treat scoliosis; one without the limitations associated with traditional treatments. And now I'm proud to be able to use my knowledge, expertise, and talent to remove the limitations that would otherwise restrict possibilities for my younger patients.

The approach we take with our patients here at the Scoliosis Reduction Center does not impose limits on what's possible for our patients. Devices like the ScoliBrace® give us a chance to truly improve the lives of young people and reduce the number of limitations they may have on their futures. When this type of bracing is done in conjunction with chiropractic care, therapy, and exercise, patients see results and improvements quickly. In fact, most of my patients notice results within two weeks of starting treatment!

Real Scoliosis Correction Is Possible!

Traditional TLSO braces like the Boston Brace and Milwaukee Brace represent technology from another era. They have a chance at minimizing the progression of a curvature, but will not actually produce a correction. They're also cumbersome, ugly, and limiting in ways that today's adolescents will just not tolerate. But the ScoliBrace® is an entirely different technology that takes the best of the old and combines it with the latest innovations in treating scoliosis.

Many patients and parents come to me with the limited belief that it's only possible to manage scoliosis. It never occurs to them that a more modern approach could actually provide dramatic scoliosis correction! That's why I'm thrilled to do what I do. Here at the Scoliosis Reduction Center, we believe that the best results happen when we treat patients who have a 3-D condition in a 3-D manner. The ScoliBrace® is a big part of that approach.

Five Facts about Physical Therapy for Scoliosis

I believe a proactive approach to scoliosis gives patients the best chance at stopping the progression of their spinal curvatures. The traditional treatment approach emphasizes observation and inaction. But this only serves to allow scoliosis to continue its progression until the point when surgery is recommended as the only viable option.

Being proactive about scoliosis means considering alternative treatments. The chiropractic-centered model puts patients back in the driver's seat of their own health and recovery. But it requires time, effort, and commitment. Not only does this approach entail scoliosis-specific chiropractic adjustments, but it also includes exercise, corrective bracing, and physical therapy.

I would like to spend some time focusing on physical therapy for scoliosis. I've found that some misconceptions exist regarding the usefulness of therapy when it comes to treating scoliosis, and I field numerous questions regarding its effectiveness. The fact is that physical therapy for scoliosis is a cornerstone of the chiropractic-centered model. Without it, treatment would not be nearly as effective. But when patients receive support specifically designed for them—and they're willing to put forth a courageous effort—it is one of the keys to halting and even reducing abnormal spinal curvatures.

Let's take a look at some of the facts about physical therapy for scoliosis.

#1—Scoliosis-Specific Physical Therapy Is Different from General Physical Therapy

When you think about the typical physical therapy program, activities like sit-ups, pelvic tilts, and resistance band training come to mind. Normal physical therapy generally includes manual therapies like stretching, massage, and strength training, all designed to remove restrictions on movement and increase mobility. Of course, each patient's physical therapy regimen is determined by the type and severity of condition they're working to overcome. Therefore, the exercises recommended to those recovering from a sports-related knee surgery, for example, are different from those that would be prescribed to someone who hurt their neck or back in a car accident.

When it comes to scoliosis, recommended physical therapy programs cater to each specific patient. And they differ from what you might expect from a typical physical therapy program. This is why generic physical therapy practices aren't effective for scoliosis. In order for therapy to have a positive impact on the scoliosis patient, it must be administered by professionals who understand scoliosis-specific exercises and therapeutic techniques. Otherwise, patients could experience more harm than good.

#2—Scoliosis-Specific Physical Therapy Is More Intense and Condensed Than Typical Physical Therapy

In order for physical therapy to be most effective in the treatment of scoliosis, it needs to be approached with greater intensity and a shorter duration. A slow, gradual path through therapy may be helpful for other types of conditions or injuries. But because scoliosis is a complex condition that progresses over time, therapy benefits considerably by ramping up the intensity.

By condensing the time frame and increasing the intensity of therapy, it's possible to overcome the progressive nature of the condition. This may sound intimidating, especially for anyone who has experienced a demanding physical therapy program in the past. However, it's not painful, and we don't push patients beyond their individual abilities to handle treatment. We simply provide more therapy over a shorter period of time so the condition can respond most favorably.

#3—Physical Therapy Is Appropriate for Mild, Moderate, and Severe Cases of Scoliosis

Whether a patient's scoliosis is mild, moderate, or severe, physical therapy is a crucial component of treatment. Naturally, the type of therapy prescribed for someone with mild scoliosis would be different from that prescribed to someone with a more severe form of the condition. Nevertheless, physical therapy for scoliosis is one of the critical pillars of a comprehensive treatment plan.

#4—Physical Therapy for Scoliosis Can Be Prescribed to Patients of Any Age

From infants to fully mature adults with scoliosis, physical therapy should be considered as a vital form of treatment. The type and intensity of therapy differs from patient to patient, and we take each person's age into account when developing a treatment plan. However, for the majority of patients, there's no age at which some type of physical therapy is inappropriate for treating scoliosis.

#5—Physical Therapy for Scoliosis Should Be Done as Part of a Larger, Comprehensive Program

By itself, physical therapy for scoliosis is marginally effective. But when it's combined with scoliosis-specific chiropractic, exercise, and custom bracing, it can provide patients with increased strength, mobility, and function. All these different modalities of treatment work together to give patients the best possible chance of halting the progression of their spinal curvatures.

Physical Therapy for Scoliosis—A Key Component of Treatment

The most common treatments for scoliosis require patients to take a passive approach. Watching and waiting, squeezing bracing, and surgery are all recognized as part of the standard, traditional approach to care. But I believe the best results are only possible when patients are proactive. That means seeking out alternative treatments like those offered here at the Scoliosis Reduction Center. Physical therapy may seem challenging, or even counterproductive, if you're accustomed to the traditional model of treatment. But it is, in fact, a critical element of addressing the condition.

Different Scoliosis Treatments, Different Results

When researching scoliosis treatments, people typically discover that there are two schools of thought. On one hand, there's the traditional, well-established orthopedic method. This type of scoliosis treatment is based on a conservative, reactive approach that involves observation, bracing, and, eventually, surgery.

On the other hand, there's the chiropractic-centered approach to scoliosis treatment. This approach is much more proactive, and it involves scoliosis-specific chiropractic care in addition to exercise, physical therapy, and specialized, corrective bracing.

Obviously, I'm biased toward the chiropractic-centered approach. I've devoted my life and profession to this type of scoliosis treatment, and the positive results my patients have achieved speak for themselves.

However, I think it's useful to compare the two scoliosis treatments so patients and parents can decide what's actually best for them and their specific situation. I believe that the people who are affected most directly by scoliosis should have access to the latest knowledge and insights. Being empowered with accurate information helps patients and their families proceed accordingly, regardless of the type of scoliosis treatments they select.

Diagnosing Scoliosis

Diagnosing scoliosis is the first step toward treating the condition.

Traditional Treatment

Patients may be screened in school or elsewhere using the Adam's forward bend test, or they may visit their doctor complaining of symptoms. The presence of the condition is typically confirmed using an X-ray, and a Cobb angle measurement is taken.

Chiropractic-Centered Treatment

Diagnosis is much the same as traditional treatment. However, I will look at multiple X-rays to determine the size and nature of the abnormal curvature in three dimensions. Because I focus on scoliosis, I'm able to learn quite a bit about the individual's condition from viewing X-rays and scans in addition to speaking with the patient directly. This helps me craft a treatment plan that's custom designed for that specific patient.

Goals of Treatment

I believe every doctor would agree that the smaller the curve, the better.

Traditional Treatment
Success is achieved whenever a patient's curve does not progress to surgical levels. The goal isn't to improve the condition, but to avoid allowing it to get to the point where surgery would be considered necessary.

Chiropractic-Centered Treatment
Our goal at the Scoliosis Reduction Center is to reduce the curve as much as possible. Success, for us, is achieved when we're able to help patients achieve real, measurable reductions in their spinal curvatures.

Observation
Most traditional treatment methods rely on a watch-and-wait approach.

Traditional Treatment
Once the condition has been diagnosed, most conventional doctors will recommend observation instead of action. They want to see what will happen with the spine in terms of the curvature's progression.

Chiropractic-Centered Treatment
Honestly, I don't believe there's much value in the watch-and-wait approach. To me, a diagnosis of scoliosis should spur action. The sooner we can start working with a patient, the more likely it is that they can experience relief and reduction.

Scoliosis Bracing
Braces are common to most forms of scoliosis treatment. There are some key differences to note, though.

Traditional Treatment
Adolescents are typically fitted with a Boston Brace or Milwaukee Brace. These braces have been around for decades and have not changed much over the years. Patients are directed to wear these cumbersome braces for eighteen or more hours each day. They work by squeezing the spine to try to stop the progression, but they don't incorporate critical strengthening and stabilizing.

Chiropractic-Centered Treatment
I also use bracing technology in my chiropractic-centered approach. Crucially, our braces are much different from traditional apparatus. They're designed specifically for each patient (as opposed to being mass-produced). Furthermore, they push the spine in a corrective, three-dimensional manner, versus squeezing the spine in a manner that limits function.

Scoliosis Exercises
Staying physically fit is an important component of a scoliosis treatment plan.

Traditional Treatment
Most conventional doctors will not recommend exercises designed to strengthen the spine and the surrounding muscles. In fact, they may actively discourage patients from engaging in any kind of exercise or physical fitness regimen. Traditional bracing apparatus also make it very difficult for patients to exercise or maintain their fitness levels, and may actually lead to weakness due to the squeezing effect they're designed to have.

Chiropractic-Centered Treatment
I believe exercise is a cornerstone of recovery and reduction for scoliosis patients. Scoliosis-specific exercises help patients reduce their

curvatures, gain strength and improve mobility. I also recommend that young patients participate in sports and other activities that involve body movement. Staying active makes the body stronger and more agile, which aids the healing process tremendously.

Physical Therapy

Physical therapy for scoliosis works in concert with exercise, bracing, and chiropractic care to reduce curvatures, build strength, and improve function.

Traditional Treatment

Physical therapy is rarely recommended. It simply does not fit within the conventional watch-and-wait approach.

Chiropractic-Centered Treatment

Like exercise, scoliosis-specific physical therapy is a fundamental component of chiropractic-centered scoliosis treatment. We use different specialized pieces of equipment, such as the scoliosis traction chair, in addition to a wide range of modalities that mobilize the spine into a corrected position. This type of physical therapy works to reverse scoliosis by creating a mirror image of the condition. Of course, each patient needs their own custom-designed physical therapy approach in order to achieve positive results. Here at the Scoliosis Reduction Center, we do exactly that.

Scoliosis Surgery

Conventional wisdom says that surgery is ultimately the only effective treatment method for scoliosis.

Traditional Treatment

Under the conventional model of scoliosis treatment, all paths eventually lead to expensive, invasive surgery. All the watching and waiting involved in this approach only ensures that the spinal curvature will progress. This leads patients to the point at which surgery becomes "necessary." Recovery from surgery becomes a lifelong pursuit, even if the scoliosis curvatures have been reduced.

Chiropractic-Centered Treatment

This is where my approach differs from the traditional treatment model most dramatically. Everything I do as a scoliosis chiropractor is meant to help patients improve so they can *avoid* surgery.

See the Difference?

These two scoliosis treatments both promise results. But I believe strongly in the chiropractic-centered treatment method. Yes, I'm biased, but my patients have achieved results that back up everything I believe. Traditional scoliosis treatments are well established. But that does not mean they're superior. Far from it.

How to Find a Doctor

This book has been all about delivering a message of hope for those affected by scoliosis. As you have read, the chiropractic-focused approach to scoliosis treatment represents a much more hopeful path forward than the traditional, surgical approach.

In my view, watching and waiting as a curve progresses is not a hopeful or positive way to treat scoliosis. But the chiropractic-focused model of treatment is different. It prioritizes taking action, and it puts the patient at the center of their own healing process. It comes with a tremendous amount of hope, too, because it provides an alternative for patients who may have resigned themselves to lives limited by their condition.

Simply put, the approach I take to treating scoliosis is extremely hopeful, but it requires patients and parents to take action. The sooner you can get started treating scoliosis, the sooner you can begin to see improvements. So, how can you begin to take the necessary steps toward healing?

You have given yourself knowledge and hope by reading this book, so you are well on your way to healing already! Now it is time to seek treatment from a qualified professional or network of providers. Finding a scoliosis doctor can be tricky, though, especially since the internet is riddled with misinformation and confusing claims about what you can expect.

Thankfully, serious standards of chiropractic-focused scoliosis treatment exist. Once you know what – and whom – to look for, you can feel confident moving forward with your care.

Why Certifications Matter

My practice here at the Scoliosis Reduction Center has become quite well known and highly regarded. That's mostly because my staff and I have been able to work with patients to produce consistent, positive results. Word has spread around the globe, and I'm proud of the fact that the treatments I provide have become so highly sought after.

There are concrete reasons why my practice has become so successful, and most of them have to do with the training I have received, and the accompanying certifications I have earned.

Patients and parents know they can trust me and my methods because they see the certifications I have earned from the most reputable scoliosis organizations in the world. These are so much more than just pieces of paper; they represent countless hours of training, education and practice.

These certifications (and the expertise behind them) are what set me apart from other chiropractors. You see, general chiropractors may be technically qualified to treat people who *have* scoliosis. But that doesn't mean they have all the tools, knowledge and options to treat scoliosis, itself. It may seem like a subtle distinction, but it's incredibly significant.

To illustrate this, imagine that you have a heart condition that requires treatment of some kind. Yes, you could make an appointment with a general practitioner, but ultimately you would visit a cardiologist who has received specific and special training related directly to conditions of the heart. Sure, your general practitioner could treat you, but they would not be able to provide the specific, targeted type of care you require.

Also consider the types of scoliosis doctors who operate within the traditional orthopedic treatment ecosystem. Scoliosis surgeons, for example, are specialists who have undergone years of training – and have received specific certifications – that qualify them to treat scoliosis. Although my goal is to prevent patients from undergoing the traditional, surgically focused approach to treating scoliosis, it's important to recognize that the highest levels of care are provided by those who have devoted themselves and their practices to the treatment of the condition. These scoliosis-specific doctors have spent their careers mastering scoliosis surgery, and they have the certifications to prove it.

When you look for a chiropractor to treat your scoliosis, it is just as important to find a provider who is focused on scoliosis to treat you. Certifications will tell you what you need to know in this regard.

My Certifications

I am happy to work with patients who come to Florida to receive treatment at the Scoliosis Reduction Center. Patients can come to me with the knowledge that they will receive fully comprehensive conservative scoliosis care, utilizing several different modes of treatment. I am capable of offering such a high level of care through various modalities because of the certifications I have earned, which include:

CLEAR Scoliosis Institute – Intensive Certification

The CLEAR Scoliosis Institute was founded in 2000, and is the leading institution in the field of chiropractic-focused scoliosis care. In addition to being fully certified by CLEAR, I am also a CLEAR instructor and Chairman of the organization's board. The CLEAR Scoliosis Institute ensures that its providers treat scoliosis using specific, tested standards of care.

https://www.clear-institute.org/clear-certification

Parker University – Digital Motion Certification

This certification qualifies me to analyze the motion of the spine on plain film and in X-Ray Motion Studies (DMX). If this is needed, this type of analysis allows me to interpret findings in such a way that I can achieve better results for my scoliosis patients.

ISICO – World Master Certification on Scoliosis and Spinal Deformities

I participated in a one-year course – and was part of the very first graduating class – to receive this certification. The course brings providers up to date with the current science regarding conservative treatment and qualifies them to determine risk factors, pathologies and underlying causes that influence treatment decisions. Furthermore, it covers all the major conservative treatment processes in the areas of therapy, exercise and bracing, providing insights into the pros and cons of each one.

https://www.scoliosismaster.org

SEAS – Advanced Certification

SEAS, which stands for "Scientific Exercise Approach to Scoliosis," describes self-corrective exercises specific to scoliosis. A basic certification and advanced certification are offered; I have both. Self correction is the process through which a patient is taught a series of movements designed to place their spine in a corrected position while performing other activities. When patients use these exercise techniques and movements, the muscles that help with the reduction and stabilization of scoliosis become stronger.

https://www.clear-institute.org/blog/s-e-s-scientific-exercise-approach-scoliosis-exercises-features/

Pettibon System – Advanced Certification with Functional Neurology

The Pettibon System is a chiropractic technique focused on spinal correction using therapy, tractions, exercises and chiropractic adjusting with the goal of restoring normal spinal position. In addition to completing advanced training for the Pettibon System, I am also a certified instructor.

https://pettibonsystem.com

ScoliBrace Certification

The ScoliBrace corrective brace system is different from traditional bracing apparatus: Not only does it stabilize scoliosis; it reduces it. These braces are custom designed precisely for each individual patient using specific measurements in concert with a provider's expertise. I am certified to prescribe this brace and customize it for each patient. Additionally, I am certified as a ScoliBrace Trainer in North America, where I am the leading provider of them.

https://www.scolicare.com/scolibrace

Max Living – Level 2 Core Chiropractic Certification
MaxLiving is an organization that was founded to transform lives through chiropractic care. My MaxLiving certification focuses on the correction of segmental misalignments in addition to spinal correction, which is the process of attempting to restore normal spinal alignment in all planes. I developed the entire process, and have served as lead instructor since 2009.

https://maxliving.com

My certifications separate me from other providers and show patients that I am able to treat scoliosis comprehensively using multiple techniques. Having all of them gives me the ability to expertly assess patients, develop treatment programs, deliver custom braces, prescribe exercises and provide chiropractic adjustments. When patients see me, they know that they are in good hands thanks to these certifications.

But what if you are a patient or parent who cannot access the Scoliosis Reduction Center?

The Power of Co-Managed Care
It may seem like you are stuck between a rock and a hard place: You know that conservative, chiropractic-focused treatment of scoliosis is effective, yet you cannot find providers in your area who have earned all the certifications I listed above. What do you do?

The answer is co-managed scoliosis care.

Although it may be impossible for a patient to receive 100% of their scoliosis care from me, they can still receive life-changing care by co-managing the condition with a local doctor. You may be asking, "how does this work?" The patient can receive treatment from me for a short time – something we call "intensive care" – and then move on to co-managed care, which allows me to work in conjunction with doctors who have some of the appropriate certifications. This way, patients can feel confident about their care, knowing that the initial decisions made regarding their condition are based on the absolute top level of conservative scoliosis treatment.

Many of my patients come to see me on occasion, but they also see providers in their local areas who have one or more of the certifications I have mentioned here. Together, we provide a comprehensive care program for each patient.

It all comes down to doing one's research and ensuring that the providers they select have the certifications necessary to provide what they require in terms of conservative treatment. When a patient or parent is aware of the certifications that matter, they can discern between chiropractors who focus on scoliosis and those who offer general care with no scoliosis focus.

Any doctor who focuses on scoliosis should be willing to co-manage with the patient's local doctor. The best doctor that can co-manage your scoliosis would be one who received some of the certifications above. When patients and parents co-manage care with providers who are certified in one or more of the areas I have discussed here, they can rest assured knowing that they are on the right path. Moreover, patients who are aware of these important certifications can avoid some of the less-than-qualified practitioners who have made themselves "internet famous" by building fancy websites that feature big promises. These providers may make a lot of money and seem like experts, but they rarely have the certifications to offer the type of care that will actually strengthen the spine and reduce abnormal curvatures.

Finding a scoliosis doctor may seem daunting, but the process doesn't have to be difficult. Providers who are certified through the organizations and programs I've highlighted in this section can offer conservative, effective treatment in their specific areas of care. Working together, they can give you more than just scoliosis hope; they can help you achieve healing.

Reasons for Hope with a New Approach to Treating Scoliosis

My Scoliosis Story: Revisited

SCOLIOSIS IS A CONDITION that's affected me personally and has had a considerable impact on the people who mean the most to me in my life. I've always had an interest in medicine; I once dreamed of becoming an MD. But circumstances—or fate, if you will—led me to become a leading scoliosis chiropractor. Thank goodness my life turned out this way!

I'm proud to do what I do, and I'm grateful for the opportunity to share my knowledge and expertise with people like you. My practice has helped countless individuals find hope and relief, but it has also helped me appreciate the unique and amazing individuals who have passed through the doors at the Scoliosis Reduction Center. I love doing what I do, and I hope that's come through clearly in this book.

My scoliosis story is one that's led me to the point at which I have influence over how people see and treat the condition. It's a huge responsibility, but it's one I'm happy to take on. Every day I get to work with patients is a day that I get to see what true hope looks like on the faces of the individuals I treat. I would not trade that for anything!

I want to thank you for taking the time to be a part of my scoliosis story. But my story isn't finished yet, and neither is this book!

I have a long way to go to ensure that my message of hope and healing reaches as many people as possible. To that end, I will continue to practice as a scoliosis chiropractor, helping those who come to the Scoliosis Reduction Center for treatment. I will also continue to develop and enhance my skills. As you know, the world is changing faster than ever before, and keeping up with the latest technology and techniques requires a diligent approach. I'm up to the challenge!

By continuing to learn and enhance my skill set, I will be able to help more people and provide the best possible information to those who are interested in my approach to scoliosis treatment. I will also continue speaking and writing about scoliosis. Doing so takes me around the world, but it also keeps me grounded here at home, in Florida, where my practice is located.

I'm happy to know that you're now a part of my scoliosis story. I appreciate you taking the time to not only read through these pages, but to also open your mind to possibilities of treatment that you may not have been aware of before. Most of all, I'm happy to know that my message of healing and hope has resonated with you.

Before I conclude this book, I want to leave you with some more facts about the contrasting choices scoliosis patients and parents of those with scoliosis must make. To me, the choice is clear. But I think it's important to reiterate the basic facts surrounding the types of treatments that are available today.

Three Reasons Why the Traditional Approach to Treating Scoliosis Is Outdated

The traditional approach to treating scoliosis isn't going anywhere anytime soon. But that doesn't mean it's the gold standard for treatment. In fact, I would argue that the traditional model of treatment is outdated compared to the chiropractic-centered approach.

Why? Here are three reasons:

#1—Advancements and Improvements Are Rarely Made

Certainly, there are things in this world that are so well defined and classic that they stand the test of time without changing. The sport of baseball, for example, is played essentially the same way it has been played since its invention nearly two centuries ago. It's perfect the way it is, just like classic designs for certain cars could never be improved upon.

Medicine is different, though. The more science discovers about the human body, the more we're able to improve and enhance the way we treat certain conditions, like scoliosis. To me, helping patients is easier and more effective when I can stay on the cutting edge of conservative chiropractic care for scoliosis. But the traditional approach to treating scoliosis has remained virtually unchanged for decades.

Take the Milwaukee and Boston Braces—the designs that are used today in the twenty-first century are the same ones, more or less, that were used fifty years ago. And that's not because they're perfectly designed. It has more to do with a reluctance to provide the type of care that might upset the status quo of traditional treatment.

The traditional approach to treating scoliosis is basically the same as it was years ago, in spite of advancements that could transform the way people cope with the condition. And it will probably remain the same for decades to come, or for as long as practitioners of traditional medicine benefit from this approach.

#2—It Is Not Effective

Scoliosis progresses. That's its nature. And yet the traditional model and approach to treatment watches and waits as the progression continues. No abnormal spinal curvatures have ever corrected or reduced this way. Surgery *can* stabilize the spine (and may reduce spinal curvatures), but that happens while introducing harmful complications and side effects. Modern medicine should be, at the very least, effective. Traditional conservative scoliosis treatment approaches tend to not be effective, and can lead to surgery.

#3—It Keeps People from Living Their Ideal Lives

The traditional approach to treatment is far from patient-centered. It asks patients to sacrifice years of their lives in order to watch, wait, and observe. It fits young people with cumbersome, awkward braces that contribute to social anxiety and prevent them from participating in beloved activities. Essentially, the traditional approach to treating scoliosis can lead to a life of limitations. I know we can do better than that!

Three Reasons Why the Chiropractic-Centered Approach Is the Present and Future of Treatment

I'm a hopeful person. I'm also a people person, which means that I get a lot of energy and inspiration from being around others. But I'm most delighted by my experiences with my scoliosis patients. They're inspiring and hopeful, and they're at the center of everything I do as a scoliosis chiropractor.

I know that my approach is effective because I see the results with my own eyes, and I hear the relief in the voices of my patients. There's absolutely no doubt in my mind that I'm providing the path of treatment that's the most appropriate choice for people today, but which is also the best choice for scoliosis patients in the future.

Why? Here are three reasons:

#1—It's Patient-Centered

I believe that patient-centered care is the future of medicine. Yes, there seems to be a trend toward impersonal, institutional care that places the patient on the margins. But I see a change coming. People are becoming frustrated with the system and its insistence that they aren't important. Medical providers and institutions will one day have to realize that putting the patient first not only is good medicine, but also is the best way to do business.

If this is the case, we're well ahead of the curve here at the Scoliosis Reduction Center. Our patient-centered approach makes us unique these days, but it's also what makes us so successful. When people hear about what my staff and I are capable of doing to help patients, they can't wait to tell others, which is why people from around the world seek us out. Our patient-centered approach is what attracts others to the Scoliosis Reduction Center now, but it's also the future of medicine.

#2—It Is Effective

If the goal is to stabilize curvatures, my approach works very well. If the goal is to reduce abnormal curvatures, my approach has also been shown to be quite effective. If the goal is to avoid surgery, there's no better approach than the one I take in my practice as a scoliosis chiropractor. It may not happen overnight, but because my approach is so effective, I believe it will become the standard one day.

#3—It Helps People Live Their Best Lives

When I was young, I couldn't participate in the sports and activities I loved. I had to miss significant chunks of school. My migraines kept me from living my best life until I received transformative chiropractic treatment. I see scoliosis patients who are told that they must limit themselves and exclude themselves from certain activities or events. It hurts me to know that they have to go through something so similar to what I experienced when I was younger.

Through the chiropractic-centered approach to scoliosis treatment, people are able to work through their conditions in ways that brings real improvement, real hope, and real healing. They're able to participate in life in ways that traditional treatment tends to prevent. Most importantly, patients who receive this type of treatment get the chance to live the biggest dreams of their lives.

THANK YOU FOR READING!

Thank you for reading this book. As I stated previously, my story—and the story I want to tell with this book—aren't over yet! There's much more work to do to spread this message of healing and hope.

To learn more about how you can be a part of this story, I invite you to reach out to the Scoliosis Reduction Center. We're located in beautiful Celebration, Florida, but our doors are open to people from all around the world. Visit our website at scoliosisreductioncenter.com or give us a call at 321-939-2328 for more information.

Made in the USA
Coppell, TX
21 April 2021